The Memoirs of Allen Oldfather Whipple

The man behind the Whipple operation

D0865173

Edited By

Samir Johna, MD, FACS
Assistant Professor of Surgery
Loma Linda University School of Medicine
Attending Surgeon, Southern California Permanente Medical Group
Fontana, California

Moshe Schein, MD, FACS, FCS (SA)
Professor of Surgery
Weill Medical College of Cornell University
Attending Surgeon, Bronx Lebanon Hospital Center, New York.

tfm Publishing Limited
Castle Hill Barns
Harley
Nr Shrewsbury
SY5 6LX
UK.

Tel: +44 (0)1952 510061; Fax: +44 (0)1952 510192
E-mail: nikki@tfmpublishing.co.uk; Web site: www.tfmpublishing.co.uk

Design and layout: Nikki Bramhill
First Edition: May 2003

ISBN 1 903378 14 1

Printed by Ebenezer Baylis & Son Ltd., The Trinity Press, London Road, Worcester, WR5 2JH, UK.

Tel: +44 (0)1905 357979; Fax: +44 (0)1905 354919.

Dedication

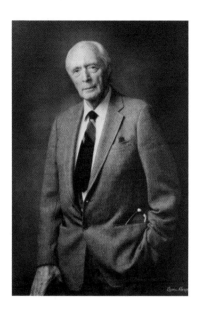

We would like to dedicate this book to Dr Richard Bing, Allen Whipple's son-in-law. He was born in Germany in 1909 to a "musical family" and began composing works of his own at the age of 6. Bing graduated from the Universities of Munich and of Berne. While a research fellow, working on cell cultures at the Carlsberg Laboratories in Denmark, Bing met Alexis Carrel (1873-1944) and his co-worker, Charles Lindbergh (1902-1974), who attended a congress in Copenhagen. Lindbergh and Carrel invited the young Bing to spend a year at the Rockefeller Institute in New York. In 1936, he became a Fellow at the Rockefeller Foundation, where working under Carrel motivated him to continue his studies on the heart and circulation. Later, after a year of internship at the Presbyterian Hospital in New York City, he met Dr. Whipple's daughter Mary who was to become his wife. In 1943 Bing was appointed Associate Professor of Surgery and Assistant Professor of Medicine in the Johns Hopkins Hospital, where he established cardiac catheterization laboratories to perform pioneering research with Alfred Blalock (1899-1964) and Helen Taussig (1898-1986). In 1969 Bing became a Professor of Medicine at the University of Southern California until he retired in July of 2002. His achievements there include high-speed cinematography of coronary vessels and studies of the chemistry of the heart after a heart attack. Richard Bing has served in the U.S. Army Medical Corps and has spent time in Germany following the World Wars helping to rebuild West Germany's cardiology program. He received wide recognition as a musical composer of more than 250 works.

Acknowledgements

We have been most fortunate in having the tremendous support of the Whipple family, more so by Richard Bing, John Bing, William Bing, Judy Tasker, Allen O. Whipple III, Richard Allen Hess and their families. Many thanks to Stephen E. Novak, Head of the Archives and Special Collections, Augustus C. Long Health Sciences Library of Columbia University, NY, his archivist Robert A. Vietrogoski, and his library assistant Henry Blanco, for their invaluable assistance in collecting data used for the footnotes. We wish to thank our publisher Nikki Bramhill at tfm publishing limited, UK, who helped us to make Whipple's work see the light.

The Editors

Contents

Foreword

On January 18th 1999, one of us (Samir) attended a course at the "Hernia Institute" of Freehold, NJ. During lunch Dr. Ira M. Rutkow, one of the two instructors and a famous surgical historian, learned that Samir is a Nestorian from Iraq. "Do you know that Dr. Whipple had written a book about the Nestorians and the role they played in the history of medicine?" he exclaimed. It was there and then that Samir became interested in the history of medicine. After reading Whipple's book he realized that Whipple had put so much effort into unravelling many facts that may not be important for the average physician today, but was certainly very important for a small ethnic minority, the Assyrian Nestorians, who are still struggling for existence in their homeland.

Writing a short biography of his, Samir thought, was the least he could do as a tribute to Whipple's contributions not only in the field of surgery but also in the field of medical history. As always, the most difficult part was where to start. Samir started with Stephen Novak, the Head of the Archives and Special Collections, Augustus C. Long Health Sciences Library of Columbia University, New York. He provided a lead to one of the surviving members of the Whipple family, Dr. Whipple's son-in-law, Dr. Richard J. Bing. After a search on the World Wide Web, Samir was able to locate Dr. Bing who, ironically, lives only 50 miles away. A few days later Samir visited him at his residence, which also serves as a small museum for the Whipple family. Amongst other things Dr. Bing showed Samir, were the unpublished memoirs of Allen Oldfather Whipple.

We are honored and privileged to take upon ourselves, with the consent of the Whipple family, the task of editing and publishing this important document. Allen Whipple's original, "raw" manuscript, which we obtained from Dr. Bing was probably written during the late 1950s and early 1960s, towards the end of his life. Whipple intended it for family use only and left it unedited. To make it publishable we trimmed the manuscript to about two thirds of its original length, removing text which appeared not to possess personal, sentimental or historical importance. We divided the manuscript into titled chapters, adding a sense of chronological progress. We also provided brief footnotes in order to identify to the readers (and us) the many names mentioned by Whipple.

Finally, the editors have decided not to include their own perspective and opinions about Dr. Whipple's memoirs; this leaves the reader to form their own views.

The Editors

Highlights of the life and career of Allen O.Whipple

Who was Allen Oldfather Whipple? Whipple, described as "the 20th century's major innovator in pancreatic surgery and Columbia (University's) most famous surgeon," [1] was well known in his own time. He was chairman of the surgery department and led the surgical service at the Presbyterian Hospital in New York from 1921 to 1946. But why is a memoir primarily written for his family worth reading by others?

Whipple's memoir offers a unique view of late 19th and early-to-mid-20th century life. The child of missionaries, Whipple grew up both poor and well educated. The memoirs reveal his odyssey from Persia to America to Europe and back to Persia and the Middle East, and contain observations on such things as kite flying in Persia, working as a migrant laborer in the early 20th century (he rode the rails to save money for medical school), college life in the early part of the century, and the work of distinguished pioneers in surgery and medicine.

We all share the mores of the times in which we live; we more rarely overcome them. Whipple was sometimes moralistic (he dismissed native Americans he met on a wilderness trek because they wore odd clothes and asked him for some trifles); yet he was the first in the United States to offer an African-American a position in a department of surgery. That surgeon, Charles Drew, distinguished himself both as a surgeon and a humanitarian.

Whipple was not always a polished narrator, nor did he in general reveal directly his own thoughts or emotions. But he had a keen eye for detail, and skill at vivid description; when, for example, he observed a near fight between a young hobo and an older fellow who "pulled out a long knife and said, 'touch me and you touch steel,'" the reader is there.

Some of us are fortunate to distinguish ourselves in a single endeavor. No fewer than four areas of Whipple's life are remarkable: his contributions to surgery; to medical teaching and research; to the study of the link between Western medicine, early Arab discoveries and Assyrian scholarship, and the science of the ancient Greeks; and to the support of medicine and medical facilities, especially in the Middle East. To each of these, he dedicated a portion of his life and his work.

The Whipple operation

Nicholas Christy has observed, "Whipple's own contribution in pancreatic surgery began by accident. In 1935 Whipple was giving an amphitheater demonstration to distinguished American and foreign visiting surgeons on a patient thought to have gastric carcinoma; halfway through, Whipple discovered that the lesion was actually carcinoma of the pancreas, so he had to devise and execute on the spot the elaborate operation still in use: pancreatoduodenectomy, involving stomach, jejunum, duodenum, pancreas, and common bile duct (also known as Whipple's operation)." [1]

It is the measure of Whipple's character that this procedure, to which he lent his name, receives but little notice in his memoirs.

Contributions to surgical education

In his retirement, Whipple was far from idle. His surgical experience and dedication to surgical education were called upon when he was asked to reorganize the surgical training program at the Memorial Hospital in New York (1946-1951) and when he served as a trustee at the American University in Beirut (1941-1957). At Princeton University, he acted as an advisor to pre-med students and became a trustee of the university (1951-1963). He served as Editor-in-Chief of Nelson's Loose-Leaf Surgery for almost twenty years, and as a member of the editorial board of the *Annals of Surgery* (1932-1946). During the last part of his career, he played a key role in the work of the Iran Foundation, which was established in New York after the Second World War to help in the development of a model hospital in Iran. Whipple, more than any other American, was responsible for the plans and policies developed for the Nemazee Hospital and for the selection of its initial staff. It was opened in 1954 and later was operated as part of the new Pahlavi University Medical School. This institution has had a tremendous impact upon health services and medical and nursing education in the whole of Iran [2].

Studies of the Greek, Arab, and Nestorian contributions to western medicine

"As a child (Whipple) learned English, French, Armenian, Syriac, Turkish, and Persian; this early linguistic immersion gave Whipple a lifelong interest in the culture, religion, and medicine of the Middle East." [1]

Whipple was intrigued by how and why the "Greek Miracle" of science and culture of the pre-Christian era, which so nearly perished, was transmitted through the Middle Ages to Renaissance Europe. It is known that Greek philosophy and medicine were translated from Greek to Syriac by the Nestorian (Assyrian) schools of Edessa and Jondi-Shapor, and from Syriac to Arabic by the small, unorthodox Christian sect of Nestorians (Assyrians) who dominated these schools during the fourth to the tenth centuries A.D. But the way these schools and their associated hospitals influenced later Arab medicine was inadequately examined [2].

In 1955 Whipple was appointed by the American Schools of Oriental Research to study the sites and remains of the medical schools and hospitals that were built during the Middle Ages in the Near and Middle East. This led him to write an important monograph in the history of medicine entitled: *The Role of Nestorians and Moslems in the History of Medicine* [3]. At his death, the manuscript was complete but not ready for the press. The monograph, finally published in 1967, is a detailed account of the medical practice, medical education, and early medical schools and teaching hospitals under Islamic rule; it also included biographies of many prominent physicians who made medical contributions during that period. The work now serves as a rich and valuable reference for students of the history of medicine [2].

This endeavor, his last, pulled together the threads of his life: his early days in Persia observing his father's work with the Nestorian community there; his extraordinary grounding in the languages of the Middle and Near East; his work in medicine; and the study in his latter years of the transmission of medical knowledge from the Greeks to today.

Whipple, the man

How will Whipple's contributions be remembered? Science, as well as art, must be judged by history in the time in which it was created. The discovery of the circulation of the blood by William Harvey in the seventeenth century was as great a step in the development of modern medicine as the discovery of DNA in the twentieth century. The first steps are of as great importance as those at the top, for without pioneers, there can be no ascent [4].

Nicholas P. Christy, in the Columbia University Journal, wrote of Whipple's "balance, kindness, energy, simplicity and genuine humility, moderation, and great versatility."

Early in his life, Whipple saw four of his siblings die. Then his father died in Persia as Whipple was completing his college years at Princeton, and Whipple thought he might never complete his studies for lack of money. One of Whipple's sons was killed in an automobile accident in his sixteenth year; his remaining son, whose psychological health had been damaged during his service in the US Navy during the Second World War, died of alcoholism while Whipple was caring for him, just a few days before his own death.

No one can know the impact of these blows on his psyche, but in the face of the most difficult circumstances Whipple carried on, always demanding of himself more than he required of others. He combined a steely determination with compassion for those who, for whatever reason, were in need of help.

He had a small house on Nantucket and later in life he studied landscape painting there. Some of his works are reproduced in this volume. They are, like his life, without pretence, but they are not without charm. For much of his later years he also played the cello with great enthusiasm in amateur string groups.

One of his grandsons, having learned chess at a young age from his grandfather, remembers a game with Whipple during the last week of Whipple's life. Whipple was prouder losing a match to his grandson than he would have been had he won. They spoke of the recent death of Whipple's son, and Whipple mused: "If heaven is a place with golden toadstools and angels with harps, I'd rather go elsewhere." A few days later, Whipple, son of missionaries, himself was gone, having outlived his wife and two sons. The old Persian expression describing Shah

Mahmoud fits Whipple equally well: "He came to this life with empty hands, and so too he departed from it."

Here in these pages you will find the man, in his own words, as he writes of people, times and places that for the most part exist no more. Here is the life of a man who overcame early adversity to make major contributions to surgery, to medicine and its history, to scholarship, and to those who needed his support. Like all men, even and perhaps especially great men, he was imperfect. But we will let him, now, speak for himself.

John Whipple Bing, Ed.D.

Footnotes

1. **Nicholas P. Christy**
   http://cpmcnet.columbia.edu/news/journal/archives/jour_v18no3/faculty.html
2. Johna S. Allen Oldfather Whipple: A Distinguished Surgeon and Historian. *Digestive Surgery*. In Press.
3. Whipple A.O. *The Role of the Nestorians and Moslems in The History of Medicine*. Princeton University Press, New Jersey, 1967.
4. Personal communication from Dr. Richard Bing, March 7, 2003.

The Memoirs of Allen Oldfather Whipple

The man behind the Whipple operation

Introduction

Living is the continuous adjustment of the individual, or persona as Jung has called it, to the happenings of life. It is the happenings such as parentage, the permanence or the change in habitat and surroundings, the place and type of education and occupation, the later marriage and family life, the tempo of living with new and fantastic inventions having to do with travel, seeing and hearing, new revolutionary discoveries in science and medicine, the peaceful or war periods of existence. It is these happenings that require continuous adjustments of the persona to his environment.

Perhaps an unusual childhood in a missionary family in a foreign and ancient country, with a background of travel and early familiarity with five languages, living in many different places in this country and abroad, a professional life in a large university and hospital in a great metropolis, all during a period of some eighty years of unparalleled scientific progress and two World Wars, makes this record of making adjustments by this persona somewhat unusual and of interest to his relatives.

A persona, as Jung uses the word, is the private conception that an individual has of himself or herself, his idea of what he is and what he wants to be, and of what he wants others to believe he is. Everyone has a persona by which he thinks of himself and others, and which gives him a standard of conduct. Without it there would be no individuality, no self-respect, no self-conduct or explanation of the individual to himself.

So, writing an autobiography, if an honest one, is more or less the revelation of the persona. But no autobiography can be complete. In discussing this subject in "Burning Old Letters", a delightful essay that I heard Dr. Rufus Cole read at the Charaka Club in New York, he had this to say: "All of us, even the most simple as well as the most sophisticated, lead two lives. In one we are engaged in eating and drinking, in working and playing, in carrying on our social activities. In the other are comprehended our loving and hating, our joys and sorrows, our ambitions and disappointments, our philosophy, our religion. Of the latter aspects of our lives the world knows little, for civilized man, especially the Anglo-Saxon, has trained himself to temper his emotional reactions and to conceal his deepest thoughts and feelings. We do not exactly laugh in the wrong places, but we do not weep in the right ones.

"It is owing to this ingrained reticence that fiction is often so much more complete and interesting than biography, and especially autobiography. Writers of fiction conceal nothing; their characters have no inhibitions. Most autobiographies are unsatisfactory not only because of a disinclination to reveal the inner self, but because we often do not know ourselves, or, still more important, because the writers do not know how to tell the little they do know.

"With most of us, if we ever do reveal ourselves, our real feelings and thoughts, it is in the letters to the members of our families and to our most cherished friends. It is this self revelation in old letters that makes one so reluctant to expose them to the risk of being read by unfeeling strangers, and so insistent on their destruction".

And so this autobiography cannot pretend to be complete in any way, just a record of times and happenings in my own life and that of those near and dear to me.

Heredity and environment play such definite roles in the life of the individual, and so often they are so intimately interwoven that it is difficult to say which of these factors is the dominant one. It is certain that had I had different parents, and had not lived for fourteen years in the Middle East, my life would have had an entirely different pattern - if one at all. In reading this story of my beginnings it will make it more interesting if one keeps in mind these two factors of heredity and environment, for their effects will be evident from beginning to end.

Biography may or may not be interesting, depending upon the subject and the author, or both. Autobiography seldom is because the subject and the author are the same, and the former can never be dealt with objectively by the latter. Yet in everyone there is a suspicion of a desire to give those near and dear to him an expression of his past in relation to the present and future of the family.

If an autobiography, brief and uneventful though it be, can be limited in its reading to the relatives of the subject and author, it may serve a useful purpose in explaining the author to those in his immediate family. So intended and so written, it should be given to the family, and seldom, if ever, to an outsider. An unfortunate necessity in writing an autobiography is the constant use of the first personal pronoun. It becomes monotonous and gives a wrong impression of the author. An apology is offered for this use of the pronoun.

Chapter One

Ancestors

One cannot tell of himself without giving some outline of his antecedents and their origin. The Whipple family, spelled in different ways during the first two or three centuries of the family, originated, it is said, with Henri De V. Hipple, a gentleman of Normandy of the Vale de Suere. For his gallantry he was granted the Memorial Estates of Wraxall, and was knighted on the battlefield of Agincourt. The name Hipple was anglicized into Whipple in the time of Henry VII (1485-1509). Later the name Whipple appears in London, Canterbury and Norfolk.

Our direct ancestors settled in the town of Bocking, near the east coast of England. Twenty Whipples were christened, married or buried in the churchyard of St. Mary's Episcopal Church in Bocking. Two names are of importance to us: John and Matthew. These two brothers migrated to Ipswich in Massachusetts in 1636, from Bocking. They built the Whipple House in that town in 1638. It is still called the Whipple House, one of the finest old houses in New England, and is now the home of the Ipswich Historical Society [1]. It is furnished with some of the original furniture, as well as with antique pieces that have been donated by the Historical Society.

Matthew was our direct ancestor who lived and died in Ipswich. His great-grandson was Francis Whipple, who married Abigail Lampson. Some of the Whipples made names for themselves during the Revolution.

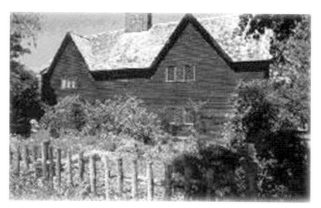

The John Whipple House.

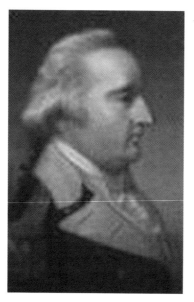

William Whipple.

John Whipple's great-grandson, William Whipple (1730-1785), who settled in New Hampshire, was one of the signers of the Declaration of Independence. Captain Abraham Whipple (1733-1819) served in the American Navy, and was commended by George Washington for bringing a valuable cargo through a blockaded harbor. The original letter written and signed by Washington is a valuable and prized possession.

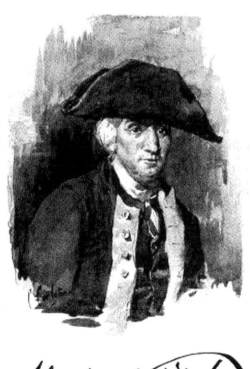

Abraham Whipple.

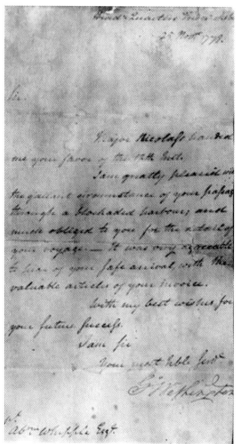

Head-quarters, Fredericksburg
25th Nov 1778

Sir,

Major Nicolas handed me your favor of the 12th [Inst?].

I am greatly pleased with the gallant circumstance of your passage through a blockaded harbor, and much obliged to you for the details of your voyage - it was very agreeable to hear of your safe arrival with the valuable articles of your invoice.

With my best wishes for your future success.

I am Sir
Your most hble servt
George Washington

Capt. Abrm Whipple, Esqr

Captain Abraham Whipple was commended by George Washington in this original letter written and signed by Washington himself.

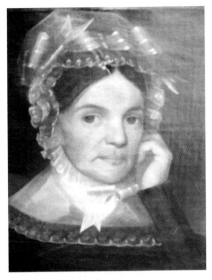

Abigail Whipple.

Francis Whipple (1705-1787) and Abigail, his wife (1709-1799), lived in Ipswich during the Revolution, and are the first of whom we have any pictorial record. Their portraits, painted as were so many in those days by unknown artists, and unsigned, are of special interest to us, not so much as portraits, but as showing certain family characteristic features: forehead, eyes, and mouth, which even in my father's and my own generation reappear in one or more members. These two portraits have since then presided on our most favored wall and will be handed down to my successors.

Of the family doings before my grandfather's generation we have little more than a genealogical record of names. My grandfather had brothers and sisters, only one of whom I knew. She was aunt Lucy who married and lived in Brooklyn. As a medical student at Columbia I made regular and dutiful visits to Jarolamen Street in Old Brooklyn to see her until she died at the age of 96. She had traveled with the family in the early 1820s when they trekked west in

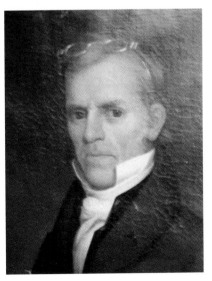

Francis Whipple.

a covered wagon across the Alleghenies. But she returned to New York later and was a passenger in the first train that went from New York to Albany.

When I knew her she was a rather pathetic old lady, with most of her faculties intact, but with some of the quirks of old age. She thought it was challenging providence to go through the subway tunnel under the East River, but her great-niece took her through it on more than one occasion without her knowing it. She had become parsimonious with a fear of extravagance, which resulted in her doing her own cooking, although she had means to employ a cook. On her 95th birthday I remember an apple pie that she had made. It was not a good pie, and I never even liked a good one, so that my exclamations of appreciation were not entirely genuine. She had become forgetful and had promised her belongings to many of her old friends and neighbors, including a set of six (empire dining) chairs to me. After the funeral, there was a distressing scene when the various promisees appeared to claim her bequests. The chairs disappeared one by one, and all that was finally left unclaimed was a dreadful Madonna of the Chair with a clock face in her middle and a glass globe over all. My efforts to bring this back to New York intact in a taxicab were not at all appreciated by my newly acquired bride, Mary. She called the janitor and asked him to take the clock away immediately, and I was in agreement.

My grandfather Francis was married to Mary Van Deeren in Putnam, Ohio, in 1840. How he came to meet this lovely girl of Dutch ancestry, of a family long resident in Basking Ridge, New Jersey, I am not informed. From Putnam and later Mt. Vernon, Ohio, where my father was born in 1845, my grandparents moved to Terre Haute, and then to Rockville, Indiana. There my grandfather owned and managed a leading dry goods store until his death in 1887. I regret that I never saw him, but some of his outstanding qualities I came to know as inheritancies in his three sons: my father, uncle Frank and uncle Lu. A gracious courtliness and gentlemanly bearing was noted by all who knew him, but a gentle reserve prevented anyone from taking advantage of his courtesy. The Whipple brow and mouth were evident in his photographs. Tall and erect, he was a gentleman of the old school.

Grandmother Whipple was the only one of my grandparents that I had the privilege of knowing when I was eight years old. She was living in Rockville, Indiana, in the Whipple house facing the town square. At that time, over seventy, she was still a beautiful woman with her lovely complexion and masses of snow-white hair. Her genial and charming hospitality as well as her natural beauty made her beloved in Rockville. One of my first recollections of her was her love of peppermint drops. She always had a supply of them in her handbag. These candies were hard and hot due to the peppermint in them. When she first gave me one I kept a straight face and did not show my dislike of it. Not wanting to hurt her feelings, I gave her the idea that I liked her candy, and so I was given a peppermint whenever I went to see her. It was not always easy to get rid of it, so I suffered slow anguish while it melted in my mouth.

Grandfather Allen, my mother's father (1805-1885), was one of several brothers of a family living in Shelbyville, Kentucky. He graduated from Center College and later from the Princeton Theological Seminary in 1836. He preached in Alabama and later, during the Mexican War, in Texas. He later married Margaret Maxwell, my grandmother, one of a remarkable family of nine children.

The Allen grandparents lived in Waveland, Indiana, when they were married. There, their three daughters, Mary, my mother, aunt Maggie and aunt Lucy were born and a son, William, who died at the age of three. The family moved to Rockville when my grandfather was called to the pastorate of the Presbyterian Church. Here the Whipple and Allen families came to know each other as intimate friends; both families were Presbyterians of the old school. The catechism, old and new, and the Bible were the only books for Sunday reading, and the latter was memorized, if not greatly enjoyed. In the Whipple family, Frank, and in the Allen family, Lucy, remained nonconformists. Although always respectful and tolerant, they were not church members, and did not look upon cards and dancing as necessarily damning.

The early childhood and adolescence of these children were permanently affected by the Civil War. Grandfather Allen, born in the border state of Kentucky, was one of the two Unionists in the family; four of his brothers joined the Confederate Army. As a result, the Allen family in Shelbyville, Kentucky, was permanently disrupted and disappeared from that town. The Whipple boys were under age until the end of the war, but many of their friends and older cousins were in the Union Army. This bitter Civil War feeling was still very strong when I first went to Rockville in 1889, and I can remember the large Grand Army of the Republic parades and the fervent speeches that were made on Memorial Day. One of the veterans who sat in front of us in church had had the lobe of his left ear shot away; this deformity held my attention more often than the sermons.

Both my parents had missionary leanings. After their marriage in July of 1872, they sailed for Persia with their classmates and close friends, the Oldfathers. The two couples were married on the same day and at the same time by Grandfather Allen in the Presbyterian Church. In mother's memoirs, "Twenty-five Years in Persia", she describes their first journey to Persia; four weeks' travel on horseback and living in tents. This, as well as the account of her later experiences in that country, is a remarkable story of tragic and amusing experiences, and should be read as an introduction to this story.

Mother's character and her faith and personality are beyond my powers of praise and description. I shall refer to some of the facets of her life as I tell of the years that follow my earliest recollections of her. She was the most unselfish person with the highest standards of living, with the most constant faith in the future, that I have ever known.

In her memoirs she tells of the births of her first two children, boys, William and Maxwell, and their early deaths from diphtheria within a week of each other. A sister Mildred was born in 1877, a beautiful child who was the pride and joy of her parents and their relatives when they returned to Rockville on their first furlough. Mother tells of their return to Oroomiah, Persia, at the time of the siege of that city by the wild Kurdish tribes from the mountains west of the city, and of father's having to stay in the besieged city while the rest of the missionaries were outside of the town in the college compound. With the raising of the siege as the result of the coming of General Wagner [2] and his Persian Army, father was able to join the family and the other missionaries.

Footnotes

1. **Ipswich Historical Society**
    Was founded in 1890 and is currently located at 54 South Main Street, Ipswich, MA 01938. The Society maintains two early Ipswich buildings of which one is called "The John Whipple House". This house was built in three stages: began in 1655 by Elder John Whipple, then greatly enlarged in 1670 by Captain John Whipple, and completed in 1700 by Major John Whipple. Most of its original timber frame is superbly fashioned of oak, chestnut, and pine which has well survived the test of time. The museum interiors contain many exceptional furnishings and decorative arts from the period of the Massachusetts Bay Colony.

2. **General Wagner**
    An Austrian General who served the Shah of Iran in the Persian Army.

Chapter Two

Early life

1881 - 1894

Father had been appointed the representative of the American Bible Society, but he maintained his close association with the mission in Oroomiah. In the latter part of August, 1881, cases of scarlet fever appeared and in the last week of that month sister Mildred came down with it and died three days later. This third tragedy, coming as it did when mother was expecting the arrival of another child, to which the little sister had been looking forward to so eagerly, was a heartbreaking experience, one that only the abiding faith of my parents could stand. Six days after the dear daughter was buried by the side of her two little brothers in the little missionary cemetery on Mt. Seir, that is, on September 2, 1881, I arrived in the Whipple home. Mother always said that my coming did more than anything to console her grief at the loss of her precious Mildred.

In 1883 father decided that it was necessary to move to Tabriz as a more central point for his work for the Bible Society. After an overland journey of five days on horseback, the family settled in the Taylor house in Tabriz, with Dr. George W. Holmes [1] and his wife and their five-year-old daughter, Mary. My parents' fifth child, Clarence, was born in Oroomiah, before they moved to Tabriz. But the next year he died of meningitis. I have a very dim recollection of my parents' grief at that time. All four of these children died of contagious diseases that today are cured with sera or antibiotics, but in those early days they were almost always fatal.

My earliest clear memory is one of playing at the foot of a tall poplar tree that stood in the lower end of the yard. Around it, mint was growing, and ever since then the smell of mint recalls that earliest clear recollection. The Oldfathers, the Holmes and other foreign families with young children persuaded mother to start a school to teach the three Rs (Reading, Writing, and Arithmetic). This she did in one of the rooms in the Taylor house. I was then four years old and can remember the first primers that were used by the youngest pupils. The first page showed a big A, and beside it was a large red apple. What the rest of the letters were illustrated with I cannot remember, but what a big red apple!

Within a month after the opening of the school, I came down with a severe headache and a fever, and soon had a full-blown case of typhoid fever. Of course mother could not act as nurse for me and conduct the school, so it folded up, much to the distress of the children and their parents. I can remember that my bed, when I was convalescing, was in front of an old-fashioned wood stove with many letters of the makers of the stove. During the weeks that I had to stay in bed I learned these letters and continued by reading lessons from the red apple primer and the second chapter of the Gospel of St. Matthew. So I learned to read by the tedious way and have never been a flash reader.

My next vivid memory is a cut that I received on the back of my head - one of my very few surgical experiences. Much bleeding, with stitches put in by Dr. Holmes, and much fuss by the two nursemaids, our Hannie and the Holmes' Munnie. The scar is still visible the barbers tell me, and would easily identify me by the F.B.I. Another early recollection is the Oldfather's yard, where there was in the summer what then looked like a large box-swing, holding four children, and in the winter, a snow hill, providing thrills aplenty on homemade sleds.

Mr. Jeremiah Oldfather, with his deep bass voice and long flowing beard, was a striking figure. As Santa Claus at Christmas he convinced us little youngsters that he had come from the North Pole. One such Christmas was made memorable by the presence of a large fir tree that my father had brought from the Caucasus for the celebration. Speaking of beards, all the men in the mission sported beavers of generous and untrimmed variety. This was a holdover from Civil War days, for one saw them aplenty in America at that time. Grandfather Allen wore a large white beard, and looked so much like Darwin, the great evolutionist, that he considered seriously of doing away with his beard so that no one could accuse him, a fundamentalist, of looking like Darwin. Fortunately he was dissuaded from doing so.

During the summer of '86 we moved to what was called the Abraham house, sharing one half of it again with the Holmes family. This house had a large flat roof with a clay fence around it that provided running room for the children and a promenade for the elders in the long evenings. It was there that I flew my first kites, which in later years gave me one of my chief summer occupations. A neighbor across from our roof, a Mr. Gerard, owned a large, rectangular concave kite with bells and large flappers on it that made a roaring sound when it was high in the air. He would have it flown in the evenings, when lanterns and banners would climb up the kite cord. To us children the kite appeared to be miles in the air.

Another next-door neighbor was Mr. Nicholaides, a Greek gentleman. He played the piano very well and gave me my first impressions of Beethoven, Mozart and Mendelssohn. An occasional caller on my father was the Turkish Consul, an enormously fat and very jovial old fellow, wearing his large red fez on his head. But the most interesting and picturesque of our European friends was General Wagner, of whom I have already spoken. He was then in Tabriz trying to get some order and discipline out of the good-for-nothing Persian Army. He was a very imposing figure in his Austrian general's uniform and decorations, and with an enormous pair of mustachios and a deep stentorian bass voice. We always knew that he had arrived when we heard him give the dervish call of Ya Hakk, Ya Hoo, on entering the gate of the yard of our house. He adored my parents and said that they were the only saintly and trustworthy people in the city. Because our cook, Karim, made such good white bread, he would rave about it and the food at our table, and usually left with two or more loaves of Karim's bread under his arm.

The summer of '87 we camped out in tents near the village of Nemitabad, some twenty miles from Tabriz. Near us was the summer camp of the Russian Consulate. The three young secretaries of the consulate came to tea with us frequently. I remember well these Russian gentlemen for different reasons: Mujnikoff because of his kindness to me in making me kites and taking me on horseback rides; Streeter because of his playing chess with father, and Count Ponafidine because of his courting and later marrying Emma Cochran. She had come to visit us from Oroomiah that summer. We knew her and her mother and brother intimately. With her and Ponafidine, a Russian Count, it was love at first sight, but neither could understand a word the other said. It became my father's delicate duty to translate the notes they sent each other. When they were together, interpretation did not seem necessary. This intriguing affair naturally brought the two camps closer together, and when the engagement was announced, the Russians gave a grand soiree, attended by all the Americans and Europeans. I remember that champagne flowed liberally, judging from the frequent loud popping and the quandary of the missionaries, all teetotallers, in not wanting to appear discourteous to their generous hosts, but at the same time not indulging in the festive wine, was a serious discourtesy. I am sure that father's tact was never more strained. The Ponafidine marriage was a very happy one, but ended tragically during the Soviet Revolution, when all the great property of Count Ponafidine was confiscated, and before he died they had little more than potatoes and a few vegetables to live on. Madam Ponafidine, who had received training as a nurse in Buffalo before coming to Oroomiah to help her distinguished brother (the great physician who built the first hospital in Persia), had been a saint to the peasants living on their estate. It was due to the help of some of them that Madam Ponafidine and her two sons were able to escape across the Bay of Finland and finally get to America. She made a great reputation with her account of their experiences during the revolution, in the articles and books that she wrote [2].

The spring of '89 was especially eventful for us children because of the preparations for coming to America for my parents' second furlough. A three-day caravan journey to the town of Julfa on the Aras River, the

Greek Araxes, between Persia and Russia, brought us youngsters our first impression of a new and more civilized country. From Julfa to Agstafa was covered in five days by post road, in troikas, and part of the time in view of Mt. Ararat. We had our first view of a railroad that took us to Batoum on the Black Sea. From that port we traveled to Odessa and Constantinople by steamer. The ride down the Bosphorus was eventful for me: I had my foot caught in a large pulley that carried the rudder chain, a very painful experience for a few minutes until my foot was extricated during which time I expressed my pain with loud cries in Turkish. This incident, when told by my parents when we reached America, with emphasis on my Turkish wails, caused me untold embarrassment.

From Constantinople up the Greek Archipelago to Athens; from there to Venice, Paris and London. My first impressions of Paris are especially vivid because the Exposition of '89 was in full swing, the Eiffel Tower and the illuminated fountains causing the greatest astonishment. Also, I was the only member of the family that could speak French, a result of my having studied that language with a M. Lampre, the Parisian tutor to the sons of the Crown Prince in Tabriz, the year before we left for America. This had given me a Parisian accent and a working conversational knowledge of the French language. Father was very pleased when the people in the pension where we were staying complemented him on my Parisian pronunciation. He encouraged me to study French in later years.

Our stay in London lasted more than a week because father had a collection of coins that he wanted appraised at the British Museum. He spoke of this to his London tailor, a Mr. Keen, who showed an immediate interest and said that he knew Mr. Sayce, the authority on oriental coins in the British Museum. What amazed me the most, when we reached London, was to find that everyone spoke English. We stayed at the Burrs - a typical English boarding house on Queen Square. Here I remember the delicious strawberries and lovely flowers that the cockney hucksters brought in their donkey carts. They soon discovered father's love for flowers and he became an easy victim of the hucksters. Queen Square with its tall plane trees and grass plots was a charming London square. I have always gone to see it whenever I have been in London, but the last two times it was forlorn with its bomb shelters and the plane trees gone.

We sailed from Liverpool on the old Anchor Line tub, the City of Rome. It took fourteen days to make the crossing to New York. Mother and I were the only members of the family to appear regularly at the dining saloon. Poor father, as was his invariable custom, went to his berth on entering the ship and did not appear until we sighted the Statue of Liberty. A sea voyage to him was anathema, and the mere discussion of an ocean voyage made him ill.

Father was detained in New York for a week by the Customs people because of his honest declaration of some curios that he had brought from Tabriz. After a hot day in the St. Dennis Hotel, opposite Grace Church on Broadway, mother and we three children took a train to Terre Haute, and from there to Rockville, where we youngsters had our first view of our aunts and uncles and grandmother Whipple, and our first impressions of the typical old Hoosier town. That was when the bicycle was still a high-wheeled affair. Horses were a necessity and the fine ones, a luxury. Mother's cousins, the Pruetts had a fine stable, some of them racers. Max, the only son, was two years older than I but because of my knowledge of Arab strain horses, I was able to hold my own end of horse tales. It was on that first day in Rockville that I was given my first peppermint candy by grandmother Whipple, and my lasting impression of her lovely character. Father's brother, uncle Frank, was as courtly as a Spanish grandee. Aunt Lucy, mother's younger unmarried sister, began immediately to be what she always was later, our good angel: a new dress for Margaret, a four-wheeled wagon for me, and a little sulky for Lucius, and all with a merry exuberant laugh, with many a mild dig at mother for her strict Presbyterian views. It was she who promptly introduced me to Tom Sawyer and Huck Finn, saying a missionary's son needed that reading more than a cat needed kittens, and she was delighted to hear me chuckling and appreciating her favorite author.

In the fall of '89, I entered the third grade of the red schoolhouse with children of my own age. In many ways I was more advanced, especially in reading and geography because of my contacts with older people and my having been in foreign countries. It was easy for me to bring home good report cards. The school was a typical small town Hoosier affair as so graphically pictured by Briggs [3] in his famous cartoons, and by Tarkington [4] in his Penrod stories. In the town there was the old swimming hole, the rail fences that we used to rattle with hoop sticks, and the town bad boy named Satan Hall.

Rockville at that time was the county seat, with the courthouse in the middle of the town square and the main stores on the four sides, with uncle Frank's dry goods store, one of the main ones, on the north side. The red schoolhouse was four blocks north of the square, and aunt Lucy's house, where we lived, five blocks west of the courthouse. She was the teacher of the fourth grade, so that she kept an eye on my doings. The incident that gave her great joy was a fight that I had with the bully in her grade. This ended in both of us having bloody noses and a black eye. Much to my relief I received nothing but praise from mother, who had been told that the bully had picked on me and had started the fight.

The bad boy of the town, Satan, was the son of the watch and clock mender, who lived on the main street leading to the town square. Satan owned a gray parrot that he had taught phrases hardly fit for a sailor. On a Sunday morning he would hang the bird's cage on the porch near the street where the people were walking to church and, as they passed, he would coach the bird from where he was hidden under the porch. The scandalous language amused some of the passers by, but it outraged others.

Father's furlough ended in the fall of '90. We left for New York in September of that year. There we met two young missionary couples who were going to Tabriz, Dr. and Mrs. Vanneman and Mr. and Mrs. Brashear. We sailed on the St. Paul, then one of the best liners in the Atlantic. Father as usual, retired to his cabin. Mother, always a good sailor, had her hands full with the three children, although Dr. Vanneman was boon companion to us as all other members of the party were out of commission. He was a Princeton graduate and had no end of fun teaching us new tricks and making us talk Spanish.

After we reached Liverpool all of us went to the Burrs on Queen Square. I remember the amazed look on Dr. Vanneman's face when a bunch of grapes was passed for dessert, and he was asked if he would have a grape or two. From London we passed to the Continent and traveled rapidly through Holland, Germany and Austria to the Black Sea, then to Batoum and Tiflis in Russia. From there we traveled by troika over the Caucasus to the Persian border. There we found the mission wagon that had been sent to take the whole party to Tabriz where we were met at the "bridge" by a large party of American and native friends. I well remember the leprous beggars, with lost fingers and noses from their disease, coming out of their caves by the side of the road and in hoarse voices called out, "For the sake of God, the Creator, have mercy on us and give us of your bounty." That was always a gruesome and repulsive sight.

Father, as the representative of the American Bible Society, had planned to go to Teheran, the capital, to continue his work. So after a week in Tabriz we packed our belongings, which we had left in that city when we went to America, and started out by carriage on the ten-day trip to Teheran. But we had traveled only one day to the village of Mianneh, when Margaret came down with a high fever making it necessary to return to Tabriz. Meanwhile word came from the Bible Society in New York telling father to stay in Tabriz. This, of course, meant an entire change of plans and a search for a house for the family. It happened that a large house with a spacious garden of some four acres was for sale. Father bought the house and part of the garden. The Mission purchased the rest for a site on which to build a Boys' School. The entire garden with the house and its front yard, the stable and stable yard, and a small orchard was a great bargain. It was all surrounded by a ten-foot wall, as was the custom in all the houses at that time.

The house contained eight large rooms, with a high porch on the south side facing the front yard. This contained a large fountain, or tank, with many goldfish in it. It was not too deep and was a great joy to us youngsters, for it was large enough for a swimming pool. South of the front yard were rooms for the servants' quarters, and north of the two-story house was the large garden with a vineyard and fruit trees in it: apricot, peach, almond and mulberry. In the garden were a variety of roses that I have never seen outside of Persia. There was a white, single, very fragrant variety growing on a rose tree fifteen feet high which when in blossom had thousands of blossoms covering the tree. Another variety was a single, yellow rose, and another had red petals inside and yellow on the outside. All of these were deliciously fragrant.

A grape vineyard covered the north side of the house, which in the fall had hundreds of clusters of small, white seedless grapes. Our gardener covered some of these with paper bags, which protected the grapes from the autumn frosts. The grapes were delicious as late as November and December. Our gardener, Mollah Kazim, grew the most amazing flowers and fruit trees. He knew how to graft the almond trees and some of them had five or six varieties of stone, or kernel, bearing fruits: cherries, plums, peaches, nectarines and apricots, which during the spring gave the most astonishing appearance with the different colored blossoms as well as the beautiful almond flowers.

Father was inordinately fond of flowers, so that the gardener, Kazim, was a great favorite. They built a conservatory at the end of father's study where there was always a profusion of geraniums, fuchsias, begonias and climbing plants, as well as a variety of tea roses. I am sure that my sister, Margaret's, as well as my love of flowers was an inheritance from my father. Although he did not know it, or preferred to disregard it, there is no doubt that Kazim was an opium eater, a common addiction with many of the Moslems at that time. I used to see him rolling his little pills, and he always took a long siesta in the afternoon.

After we bought the house and garden there were alterations and additions that had to be made. This brought in native masons, bricklayers, hod carriers and day laborers, which gave me a chance to see them at work and to observe their methods. The bricklayers made mud bricks that the masons used later in building new additions and walls. The masons had young apprentices who threw the bricks and half bricks to the masons, as they called for them in a loud chantey. The mud and mortar, as well as other building materials were carried up by the hod carriers on ladders, as the walls got higher. Some of these hod carriers were remarkably strong fellows, carrying loads as much as three hundred pounds on their right shoulders. The brick-makers made a brick mold for me and a hod on a scale for my ten years, and were greatly amused to see me work with them.

One of the masons, who worked for us in other capacities as well, had an unexplained protection against scorpions that were frequently found in the old buildings that were being demolished. When he ran into a nest of these scorpions he would reach in and pull out three or four of the venomous creatures and put them inside his shirt next to his bare skin. They never seemed to strike him, although they would attack and strike anyone else on the least provocation. He was an inveterate pipe-smoker and always reeked with the smell of tobacco. Whether this had anything to do with his protection, I am not able to say. But I do know that if scum at the end of a pipe stem is rubbed in the mouth of a snake, it will stiffen and die in a few minutes, for I have tried it on garter snakes. Some of these scorpions were wicked looking creatures, dark yellow in color, and the large ones measuring three to four inches in length. It is said that a black variety that is found in Southern Persia is much more poisonous than the yellow variety.

The large building that was made for the Boys' School on the west end of the garden adjoined our property. Some two hundred boys of all ages, mostly Armenians, came as day pupils, although about eight were boarders in a dormitory near the school building. Some of them were good athletes. Lucius and I shared a good many of their games: foot-racing, wrestling, tops and marbles. A game like marbles was played with the dried knucklebones of sheep, which anatomically were the scaphoids of the animal. These were placed in a row of ten or more in the middle of a circle six feet in diameter. From a mark six feet beyond the circle one of the larger knucklebones, made heavier with lead, was used as a missile and chucked at the row. If the one shooting knocked any of the row out of the circle, he could continue chucking from the rim of the circle. If he missed, the next player set up the row and had his try at it.

Mother instructed us in English, arithmetic, geography and history. I studied reading and writing Persian at the Boys' School. I had learned to read and write the Syriac [5] and Turkish that were the languages that our servants used. In fact, I read the Bible in Syriac before I did so in English, for our morning prayers were conducted in Syriac with the servants who were Nestorian Christians [6], and a chapter was read each morning; the servants, my parents and I reading a verse in rotation. For a year I continued my French lessons with an old Armenian, who was not too good an instructor, but he loved to repeat La Fontaine and taught me many of the fables, some of which, even at this late date, come back to me in French. The same is true of some of the poems in Persian that I learned while a boy in Tabriz.

Soon after we had settled in the new home, father bought us children a very handsome white donkey. He was our joy and delight, for we could ride him in the avenues in the garden, and he later served us, in succession, as the animal we rode to the summer camps and, on two occasions, on trips to and from Oroomiah. He was a gentle beast, although going by the name of Nebuchadnezzar; gentle until he came within sight of the female of his species, when he let out with a sonorous bray that could be heard blocks away. I have a picture of the three of us and our little neighbor, Rhea Wilson, all seated on the long Pallan, or saddle, on the donkey's back.

The summer of '89 was a very bad one because of the cholera epidemic that swept through that part of Persia. At one time in Tabriz in August more than two hundred inhabitants died in one day, and for a week it was impossible to bury the dead. I remember seeing people dying or dead of the scourge as we passed on the road to the camp where we went to get out of the city. When we passed through a village we would see corpses being washed in the village stream, and farther down the stream, water was being taken in jars for drinking and washing. The Moslem doctrine that water is purified after it has flowed nine feet, and the belief that walking under a row of Korans strung across the village street would protect one from the disease, explains the terribly rapid spread of the epidemic. By boiling all the water and eating nothing but thoroughly cooked food, none of the family or the servants contracted the cholera.

It was here that summer that I spent a good part of my time on horseback, and at first bareback, the best way to learn to ride. One of the three horses that we owned was a beautiful chestnut with a lot of Arabian horse ancestry. He was a stallion, but gentle and very well behaved. On him I had many a race with Dr. Vanneman who rode a high-spirited gray stallion that kept the doctor busy controlling him. The horses were fairly evenly matched and they gave us some very close races over the desert. The doctor was able to come to the camp after the worst of the epidemic had passed.

Mollah Kazim was an expert pigeon fancier, especially the breed of tumblers. He introduced me to the raising and flying of this kind of tumbler, which is entirely different from the tumblers that I later used to see occasionally in New York. In this country the tumbler is a nondescript flopping bird when flying with other pigeons. In Tabriz the tumbler was especially bred to bring out its tumbling qualities. Some of the finest of them had developed two extra tail-feathers, which increased the power, and check of their tumbles enabling them to tumble vertically instead of the floppy somersaults which one sees in the tumblers in America. When these birds circled and tumbled upward two or more times a loud snapping sound could be heard at quite a distance. Some of the finest birds would circle and tumble until they were almost out of sight, and yet could be distinguished from the other flocks that were flying at the same time.

Mollah Kazim made two pigeon lofts on top of the roof of the stable and procured several fine pairs of these tumblers. They soon increased in numbers, for a pair that were life mates usually produced six to eight pairs of squabs every year. It was interesting to see eggs hatch, the scrawny, naked little squabs quickly develop feathers, and to see both the parents feeding them. Most interesting was teaching the young birds after they had grown their wing feathers to fly and to keep with the older birds in the flock. This was an art in itself, for it was easy for the young birds to join another flock if it were nearby. At first we returned the young birds of our neighbor's that came down with our flock. But when one of the neighbors to whom we had returned more than one of his birds refused to return our young birds, we decided that as far as he was concerned, finding was keeping. This particular neighbor had a very fine breed of black tumbler. When one of his best young black birds came down with our flock we were careful to tie its wing feathers until it had become thoroughly at home with our flock and loft. The man was all for renewing the former agreement, but we said we could not trust him, so we kept his bird and he became one of the finest in our flock. Kazim and I spent early morning and late afternoon hours flying and training our flock of over fifty tumblers.

Another interesting occupation in the spring and summer was kite flying. The kites as they were then made in Tabriz were of various sizes and decoration, but all were of a rectangular shape, convex on the front and concave in the back, held in that shape by bow strings tied between the four to six reinforcing crosspieces of bamboo. The paper covering them was stretched over the convex surface of the kites, and the paper was decorated with medallions and corner pieces of colored paper, very much like the patterns of the Tabriz carpets. Fitted over the cords that bowed the kite were flippers of thick paper which, when the kite was in the air, rotated, making a roaring noise. In addition, the large kites had sleigh-like bells attached to the tails and side-whiskers, which added to the noise these big kites made. The tails of the big kites were always long, some of them 40-50 feet long, which gave them great stability and favored their rising at an acute angle to great heights.

There was always an east wind at night in the summer evenings, which was a cooling blessing after the hot, dry days. This was the time for kite flying, and large and small, the kites would soar over the city. The roofs of the houses were flat and provided an ideal place to start the kites flying. In the evening, after the kite had climbed several hundred feet in the air, we would thread a lighted paper lantern on the string of the kite and watch it climb to the kite. With the steady east wind, the kite would stay up until bedtime, when we would reluctantly pull it down, winding the cord-stick, gather in the long tail and put the kite away until the next evening. The flat roofs were the sleeping quarters for the servants during the rainless summer, for there was no dew and the night breeze was better than any sleeping powders. I usually slept on the porch on the north side of the house where the sunrise would waken me in time for the early pigeon flight before breakfast, and before the lessons began.

Footnotes

1. **George W. Holmes (1842-1904)**
    Born in Indiana. A physician who from 1874 was the Vice-president of the Iowa Union Medical Society. In 1883 he became a missionary physician in Persia where he also served as a physician to the Shah of Persia. Little is known of his whereabouts during the period 1883-1903.

2. **Books published by Mrs. Emma Cochran Ponafidine**
    Russia, My Home. Indianapolis: Bobbs-Merrill Company, 1931 and *My Life in the Moslem East*. Indianapolis: Bobbs-Merrill Company, 1932.

3. **Claire Briggs (1875-1930)**
    A native of Sauk County (Wisconsin) who contributed to the development of modern newspapers and contemporary mass communication. Briggs invented characters with which millions of people could identify. He portrayed the comfortable, front porch, "good old days". His cartoons were syndicated across the country and, by the 1920s was one of the most highly paid illustrators in the country.

4. **Newton Booth Tarkington (1869-1946)**
    An American author. His popular novels dealt with life in small Middle Western towns, including *The Gentleman from Indiana*, 1899; *The Conquest of Canaan*, 1905; the

28

trilogy *Growth*, 1927; *Made up of Turmoil*, 1915; *The Magnificent Ambersons* (1918; Pulitzer Prize), and *The Midlander*, 1923. *Alice Adams* (1921; Pulitzer Prize), which is considered by some to be his best novel, tells of the frustrated ambitions of a romantic lower-middle-class girl. He also wrote several amusing novels of boyhood and adolescence, the most notable being *Penrod*, 1914 and *Seventeen*, 1916. His plays include a dramatization of his own historical romance *Monsieur Beaucaire*, 1901, and *Clarence*, 1921.

5. **Syriac Script**
    Also known as Neo-Assyrian, which the Assyrians had adopted after the cuneiform script. It is originated from Aramaic. The term "Syriac" comes from the term "Asuryaya" meaning Assyrian. It is read as "Suryaya" because the letter (A) is silent. The term has nothing to do with Syria, and is by no means synonymous to Syrian. In fact, Syria is named after the Assyrian empire that encompassed the present day Syria.

6. **Nestorian Christians**
    The Assyrians who followed Patriarch Nestorios were given this name in the fourth century. In 431, the Catholic Church through the council of Ephesus, had deposed Nestorios, the patriarch of the Assyrian church, because of what was considered heretical doctrines by his denial of the complete mergence of the divine and human natures in the person of Christ. He asserted that Mary, the mother of Christ, should not be called the mother of God. His followers, the Assyrians, were since called the Nestorians.

Chapter Three

The teen years in Persia

1894 - 1896

In the autumn of '94, I was thirteen. My parents felt that I should have a more systematized education to prepare for high school when we returned to America. I was invited by Rev. Coan to live with them in Oroomiah and attend the school conducted by Miss Lincoln. When I left Tabriz for Oroomiah I traveled on horseback with Eeshoo, our faithful hostler. Father had given me a fine bay Turkoman stallion with a very fast walk and gallop. We carried little luggage, sleeping on the roofs of the caravanserais at night. Starting at two o'clock in the morning, we would travel until near noon, rest for two or three hours, and ride again until five in the afternoon. We covered the 160 miles to Oroomiah in three days, a trip that took the family five or six days to travel by the same route. It was in September then, at the height of the grape and melon season. For five cents we could get all the grapes we could eat, and for the same sum, we got long, yellow muskmelons that were incomparable in taste and texture. Our breakfast consisted of bread and native cheese, very much like Roquefort, and several glasses of tea.

The midday meal was much the same except for the fruit. The evening meal was sherval or a roasted chicken and rice, the very good fluffed rice called pilau. All our meals were eaten native style, seated on the floor or roof, without such things as knives and forks, for the very thin bread could be rolled into useable spoons and forks, the fingers doing the rest.

One of the most vivid memories of these trips across the desert was meeting camel caravans in the early dawn, and hearing the first booming of the camel bells that some of the camels carried on either side of their loads. As we came nearer the sound deepened with the slow cadence of the camels walking. The lead camel usually had no load except for the large booming bells that he carried, together with his elaborate and fancy trappings. Some of these bells were two feet tall and eight or ten inches in diameter. Walking beside the lead camel was the head cameleer, sometimes sound asleep, or he might be singing a chantey in a loud voice to be taken up by the other cameleers in the caravan. I once counted 800 camels in one caravan. That was long before the advent of motor lorries, which today have replaced the camel caravans for freight transportation. At that time there were no railroads, and it was long before motor vehicles were introduced into that country.

The camel is the haughtiest, but at the same time the meanest, animal ever tamed by man. It has a fetid breath; it moans and groans when commanded to kneel for loading and unloading, with the gutteral order of ikkh-ikkh-ikkh of the cameleer, accompanied by the taps of the driver's staff on his forelegs. I shall have more to say about the camel later in describing the Bedouins, or Bedawi as they are called in Arabic.

When I reached Oroomiah I was given a room in the Coan home that opened off their living room, and did my studying at night while Fred and Ida were playing the piano or organ, singly or in duets. I became so used to this that I found I could study better with the sound of their music than without it. This made me more familiar with classical music than ever before, and I developed a taste for that kind of music that has stayed with me ever since. Every weekday morning the Coan children, Elsie and Frank, and I were driven to the College compound, about two miles outside of the city, to attend Miss Lincoln's classes. Dr. Cochran was the medical missionary in Oroomiah. His parents were two of the first missionaries to come to that city; he was born there and knew, read and spoke the languages of Turkish, Syriac and Persian like a native, as did his close friend Fred Coan. He was a talented physician and was not only adored by both the Christian and Moslem populace, but was almost worshipped by so many of them that he had cared for, especially the wild mountain Kurds for restoring their sight with his cataract operations.

These people looked upon his restoring eyesight as a miracle, and spread his fame all over the Middle East. It was he and his remarkable work in the mission hospital that gave me my first interest and desire to study medicine.

The year before I came to Oroomiah, Fred Coan had imported the first bicycle that had ever been seen in that part of the country. The novelty of the thing had by no means worn off when he taught me to ride it. The young bucks always wanted to race against it, and were amazed and chagrined to find that they could not keep up with it. One day I had to pump up a soft tire and the group of boys and men, some of them Kurds, were astonished to know that I was giving the beast air. They called it the yale atti, meaning a wild horse.

The Oroomiah valley, coming down from the Kurdistan mountains in the west, was noted for its fertility, irrigated by the Oroomiah river, a clear stream varying in depth with the seasons. The vineyards and orchards were famous for the variety and quality of the fruit. I remember attending a feast in one of the vineyards in the autumn, where we tasted and counted 32 varieties of grapes, in all sizes from the small seedless white grapes to what they called the buffalo variety, deep purple and as large as the adult thumb. The muskmelons were equally famous, oval in shape and twelve to thirty inches long, with delicious flavor and fine texture. The native banquets, which in the summer were served outdoors in the vineyards or gardens, were gargantuan affairs with from fifteen to twenty courses. Rice cooked in several colors and flavors, but always fluffy, was the base for several varieties of mutton, ranging from an entire barbecued lamb to the skewered sheep tenderloin and several kinds of stews, flavored with different herbs, including plenty of onion and garlic. Cucumbers, eggplants and young grape leaves were the wrappings for a mixture of meat, rice and nuts, called dolmas. Both the Moslems and the missionaries considered wines taboo, but sherbets of different kinds were served. Desserts consisted mostly of sweets and fruits, and the meal was completed with many small cups of Turkish coffee, accompanied with the bubble-bubble water pipes called kalyans, or long-stemmed pipes called chebooks. One of the peculiar customs to show appreciation of the feast, which was anything but pleasing to the Americans, was loud belching at the end of the meal, while hand basins of rosewater were passed around to the guests to wash their hands, which had been used instead of forks. These meals were always served on cloths spread over the carpets, the guests in the cross-legged position.

Clement and I rode a great deal, accompanying the older members of the mission to the neighboring Nestorian villages, or on short trips to the mountains west of us. We also did a lot of work after school hours in chopping wood for the stoves that heated the rooms in the winter. We also built a dam on the river south of us, hoping to use the pond for a skating rink, but we never got the necessary skates in time. We both spoke Turkish and Syriac like natives and were thoroughly familiar with the customs of the different nationalities, so that we had no difficulty in getting along well in the country and villages. In fact we were as much amused as the natives in hearing some of the new members of the mission trying to pronounce and speak the languages.

In the spring of 1896, the second year of my stay in Oroomiah, Mrs. Cochran died of severe pneumonia. This dreadful tragedy for the doctor and the five children was greatly relieved by the Coans, such close friends, who then moved from the city into the Cochran home and I with them. This made a full house with eleven at the table. My duty at meals was slicing the loaves of bread for the large family.

In May of that year my family in Tabriz was beginning to get ready for the journey back to America. The family had now grown with the arrival in '93 of sister Mary, and in '95 of sister Eunice.

One of the difficult problems that my parents faced was what to take to America, and what to leave in Tabriz to be disposed of in one way or another. There were so many things in the house in which we had lived, so enjoyably, that had a great deal of sentiment attached to them, and with which we hated to part, but they could not be sent to America. One solution, and a wise one, was to give the house and the furniture to the mission to be used as a women's hospital. The rugs, antiques and personal belongings had to be packed in heavy cases to stand the long trip to the States. Our white donkey had died two years previously with tetanus due to a bad job of shoeing. Our Great Dane dog, Nero, we gave to one of the European colony. We had a family picture taken with the three faithful Nestorian servants, who had been with us from fifteen to twenty years. This was taken in the front yard with oleander bushes on the porch as a background. A copy of this is a prized possession.

In June we left Tabriz by carriage to Julfa on the frontier, and were "poured" on the road, as the natives call it, by a host of native, American and European friends that accompanied us to the "bridge" ten miles outside the city. We took Hannie and Eeshoo with us as far as Tiflis, where the good-byes to these dear and faithful servants were very tearful to them and to us. At the so-called hotel in Julfa, the first in Persia, where we stopped overnight before going into Russia, we noted a toothbrush in a cup on the washstand. Above it was a notice, which read: "This is for the use of our guests, no extra charge!"

Eunice was then only nine months old, and Mary only three years old, so that there was plenty of baby carrying for the men, and special duties for mother. She made good use of her situation when it came to customs inspection by the Russians. She had become very interested in a series of articles in the Century Magazine by George Kennan, describing the dreadful conditions of the prisoners in Siberia. She had two numbers that had arrived just before we left Tabriz, which she had no time to read. She knew that if these were discovered they would be immediately confiscated, and possibly get us into trouble. She carefully hid these two magazines at the bottom of the baby's diaper bag, covered with the dry articles, and opened the bag for inspection whenever the customs inspectors were carrying out their duties. But one look at the not too dry top contents of the bag quickly dissuaded further search!

From Batoum we sailed to Constanza, in Romania, and from there we traveled by train to Budapest and Vienna. These two cities were in the heyday of their magnificence, the beauty of their buildings, their museums and their opera. Vienna was having an exposition that year, and everything and everyone was in gala attire. My recollections of the elaborate exhibits are mixed with the memory of sharing the burden of carrying Mary, whose feet and interest in the whole affair gave out early. Father was especially interested in the very remarkable exhibit of Persian carpet and rugs, one of the finest that has ever been shown. This collection remained in Vienna for many years, where I again saw it in 1933.

From Vienna we traveled to Brussels and London. Again we went to the Burrs on Queen Square. While in London father took me to see his friend, Mr. Keen, who had been his tailor ever since his first visit in London in 1872. This was a typical old London firm, established eighty years before by the grandfather, and had been in High Holborn in the same building ever since. When I was in London in 1943, during the last war, I found that the old establishment had been bombed out, but had been moved nearby to Southampton Row. It was still doing business in 1960 when I returned from the Near and Middle East.

After crossing the ocean to New York we went to Rockville, where it was a blessed relief for mother to reach the old Allen home and the very willing hands of aunt Maggie and aunt Lucy. The following week we left for Duluth, Minnesota, where uncle Lu and his family lived. Father decided to settle there because of the delightful climate and the very good schools, and especially because uncle Lu had offered to give father a job in his office, a most necessary consideration as his work with the Bible Society had terminated.

Chapter Four

Life in Duluth, Minnesota

1896 - 1900

This was a new and exciting chapter in our lives, for it was a new venture in an entirely different way in pioneer country at that time. We first lived in the other half of the apartment where uncle Lu and his family were living. But we later moved to a larger house in a suburb on the shore of Lake Superior. It was a rambling old house, but comfortable and very pleasant because of the lakeshore and the woods that surrounded it. It was about four miles from the city itself, and at first the only means of getting to the city was by way of a Toonerville-like trolley. Later I purchased a Columbia bicycle from my savings and used this to go to and from school.

I was entered as a freshman in the Duluth Central High School. This was a handsome long building, occupying an entire city block, with a tall tower with a great clock near the top that sounded the hours and gave the time for miles around. At first I was considered somewhat of a freak, speaking four foreign languages, and not having come up through the grade schools. My classmates had had half a year of Latin and algebra, which I had not, so that when I began I had a lot of extra studying to do to catch up in those two subjects. But I had two very kind and able teachers who tutored me until I had caught up with the other classmates.

Mr. Custance, a former Don in Oxford University, was the teacher in Latin and he gave me a thorough grounding in that language. This proved most valuable when I went to Princeton, where I tutored in Latin for two years, helping to pay my expenses. The principal of the high school, Mr. Loman, was a Yale graduate, strict in discipline, but just and fair; I came to have a high regard for him. He was a fine speaker and interested in training some of us in debating. In my junior year, as a member of the debating team of the high school, we had contests in a number of the cities of the state.

I have referred to the bicycle. It was a great convenience as well as sport. In those days the young fellows had what they called "scorchers", with low-slung handlebars, used in racing. These with the high stiff collars that were the style were a very uncomfortable combination. Periodically on Saturdays there were century runs, when a hundred miles over rough roads, some of them thumping corduroy, made a form of exercise and physical punishment that the young men of today would not attempt. Not infrequently bicycle parties were arranged with the girls. Their long skirts and mutton leg sleeves required "female" bicycles. In those days shorts and lower extremity exposure were not common.

In the fall of '97 father bought a nine-room house, about a mile from the high school and near one of the good grade schools where the other children went to various grades. It was a comfortable house with a barn and a vegetable garden that kept the boys busy during part of our spare time.

In those days in Duluth it was customary for the boys to work in their spare time and during the summer. When I was sixteen I earned my first outside money delivering the Chicago Tribune after it had arrived on the nine o'clock train at night. This paid only five dollars a month, but later that year I was able to get an afternoon paper route with the Duluth Evening Herald that paid me twelve dollars a month. However, this took time from three-thirty to six o'clock every weekday. I had to deliver batches of papers to the downtown news stands for the first hour, and then deliver the Herald to the subscribers on the west end of town. This meant walking some twelve miles after school before reaching home for a seven o'clock dinner. The city of Duluth is built on a number of rather steep hills. In delivering the papers I rolled them, bent the rolls and threw them onto the porches of the houses as I walked by them. If I did not hit the porch, I had to climb from ten to twenty steps to retrieve the paper and deliver it on the porch. This certainly encouraged accuracy and developed it, so that I got expert at hitting the front doors of the houses. This caused no complaint, for it was a signal that the paper had arrived. This daily walk, rain, snow or shine, was the best kind of regular exercise, and I am sure strengthened a strong constitution that I had inherited from my Scotch ancestors on my mother's side. In Duluth the winters were rugged with temperatures as low as 30 below zero. But it was a dry cold and I never wore an overcoat while delivering papers; I had to be careful with nose and cheeks. On more than one occasion I was warned by a passerby to rub them with snow to prevent white spots that were beginning to appear.

After my junior year in high school I decided to go to a preparatory school in Woodland, a northern suburb, to get special training for college entrance examinations. This school went by the lofty name of Craggencroft, and had a pompous headmaster, who was a typical pedant, but an able teacher and drillmaster. At the same time he was a scoundrel for later he deserted his wife and eloped with one of the ladies of his faculty. I should be thankful to him, for he knew the Dean in Princeton and recommended me for a full scholarship, which I held during the four years I was there. By January of 1900 I was ready for the examinations that were given in June. During the next five months I worked in the County Treasurer's office as a clerk and saved enough money to pay for the first half of my freshman year. But the business of adding interminable columns of figures in making tax reports cured me of ever wanting to work in a bank or any commercial firm. One of my duties in that office was answering the telephone to people asking for information about their taxes. In the two weeks before the deadline for paying taxes the phone was especially busy. One morning an old lady appeared before the wire screen of the inquiry desk. She pushed a long ear trumpet below the screen and showed me a description of her property and asked what the tax was. By that time I was so used to answering these questions on the telephone that, without thinking, I said: "Please hold the line while I look up your tax." Fortunately, the old lady had a good sense of humor, which helped my apologies to her!

In the middle of May I had a succession of measles, chickenpox and mumps, which left me with only ten days to review the subjects for the college entrance examinations. I am sure that I never worked more consistently and with more concentration. I passed all the subjects except German Composition, and this I passed a few days after reaching Princeton. As a result of the measles and the concentrated work that I did during the ten days, I had to wear glasses. I had one experience during the attack of measles that permanently prejudiced me against homeopathy. I suppose my parents called in a homeopath because he had been the physician for uncle Lu's family. His treatment of me when I had a temperature of 104 degrees and was delirious with nightmares of vanishing water, with which I was trying to quench my thirst, was to prescribe a teaspoonful of water every hour, with a drop of some medicine diluted to the tenth decimal!

Ever since we had left Persia, father had felt that the work he was doing was not what he had consecrated his life to, and now that the family was settled and getting educated, he longed to return to the mission field and have mother and the two younger girls join him in Persia for a few years. Mother was in entire sympathy with this plan, although she realized that this would mean a separation for some time. When a call came from the Presbyterian Board of Foreign Missions for father to return to Persia, he and mother and the rest of the family were faced with a difficult decision. This was further complicated for mother by the fact that I had been entered in Princeton that fall. For those not brought up in a missionary family this would seem to be a far-fetched decision, but for my parents it was not; quite the contrary, it was an unquestioned call to duty. Hard as it was, they faced it and father accepted the call. He left us late in August. He was then fifty-five years old, in good health as we all were, and looked confidently to the future and to his return to us. We owned the house we were living in and I was able to support myself. Aunt Maggie and Hector were living with us and sharing in the household expenses, and she was giving valuable piano lessons to the girls. Of course it was mother who bore the burden of separation anxiety, but, as always, she was brave, cheerful, and always a good manager keeping the family budget clear, although many an evening meal was made up of baked beans.

Chapter Five

Princeton, New Jersey
1900 - 1904

In early September of 1900 I left for Princeton. Uncle Lu had obtained a pass for me on one of the ore boats to Detroit. From there I took a train to Trenton, and landed by trolley in Princeton on a very hot and humid afternoon, as green as any freshman in the class. A garret room at 44 Mercer Street for $2.00 a week and meals at $4.00 at the same place started me off. I had letters to two of the professors. One of them made arrangements for me to tutor in Latin that was a real help during that first year.

During the first week I met Dick Pell and Frank Cline who were more familiar with the customs and traditions of the college, and what a freshman was supposed to do, which helped me to get orientated. Later in the year I moved down to the second floor and shared a much better room with Frank Cline. Like all the classmates, I soon became familiar with the hard-boiled sophomores, or horsers as they were called. At that time, horsing or hazing the freshmen by the sophomores, was flagrant. The latter, wearing their club horde hats, gaudy and bizarre looking, were a constant menace to the lowly freshmen who had to wear small, black caps, called dinkeys. I well remember giving my high school yell at the order of a group of sophomores, as well as making love to a lamp post, and responding to the order to sing "In the Good Old Summertime" and listening to the caustic remarks about my dreadful singing voice. It paid to be submissive and to obey the orders promptly, for the freshman that balked or showed resentment was a marked victim for worse hazing later.

At times the compassionate juniors would rescue a freshman if they were passing by and thought that he was getting too much hazing.

The Sophomore-Freshman cannon-rush and cane-spree as well as other interclass contests, soon made it apparent that our class of 1904 was thoroughly capable of caring for itself. Freshman year was in many ways a deciding year for future activities: athletic, literary and social. I decided to try for the Daily Princetonian, the college daily, for it offered an opportunity to get acquainted with members of the faculty, one's classmates and the activities of the university. The men who were elected to the Princetonian Board were prominent in the class and merited distinction. When the contest began, some forty freshmen appeared, but after a few weeks the group had dwindled to twelve and then the competition really began.

I came to know two men on the faculty from whom I could almost always get a news item. One of them was Laurence Hutton [1], the well-known writer and literary critic; the other was Enno Littmann [2], a German philologist who had been imported by the Butler Expedition to decipher the early Arabic inscriptions that had been discovered in the excavations in Palmyra and Arabia Petria. Littman was one of the leading Semitic scholars in Germany, familiar with some seventeen Semitic languages and dialects. Most of the news items I got from him were dry as the squeegees that they had made from the rock inscriptions; but when the "Prince", as the Daily was called, was short of news, I could always turn in an article on the discoveries of the expedition. Professor Laurence Hutton was a delightful and charming fellow, familiar with so many of the literary figures of the day and a close friend of the great actors like Edwin Booth [3], McCullough [4], and Jefferson [5]. His library was as interesting as any that I had ever been in, for in it were the many photographs of his famous friends, and his unique collection of life and death masks. His *Talks in a Library* is one of the most interesting books that I have ever read. Seeking news and meeting members of the faculty as well as the men in the upper classes increased my knowledge and acquaintance with the doings of the university. It also kept me fully occupied outside of my studying and tutoring.

In May of 1901 I was elected to the Princetonian Board and was busy preparing for the final examinations of the year. It was then that I received a telegram from Mr. Robert E. Speer, Secretary of the Mission Board, telling of father's death from typhoid fever in Hamadan where he had been working since his return to Persia. I immediately telegraphed mother that I was coming home, and during the next few hours settled my affairs in Princeton, not expecting to return. It was a sad ending to a busy and happy year.

On a coach train I left for Chicago, but when I reached that city and the station to take me to Duluth, I discovered that I was three dollars short of the carfare. At the ticket window next to me was a typical Kentucky colonel of the old school who saw my predicament and said, "Son, here is ten dollars and my card. You can return the money when you reach home." But I was young and did not do justice to the gentleman's kindness, but said that I could get the necessary money and thanked him. I thought that I could pawn my raincoat, but the time was short and I could see no three-ball sign, so I hurriedly offered my coat to an Italian fruit dealer, was paid the three dollars and just caught the train.

Mother was brave, as always, and very dear, but I could see that she was heartbroken. Many a night I heard her sobbing, and sometimes I helped her to go to sleep by giving her a massage. She had always had a clear soprano voice and sang a great deal, but after father's death I have never heard her sing again, even in church.

Because of my college marks and the start that I had made there, as well as the help that our cousin Will Potwin promised mother, she insisted that I should return to Princeton. I got another job in the County Treasurer's office during that summer and earned enough money to help mother and to return to my class in Princeton. That fall I started with my cousin Hector, who entered as a freshman. We shared two rooms in Brown Hall. He had worked as a reporter on the Herald in Duluth and was a confirmed newspaperman, not interested in a college course, so he returned to Duluth at the end of his first term to resume his work as a reporter on the Duluth Herald.

Two happenings had much to do with my course in sophomore year. I was chosen as manager of the Robador dining club, which gave me my board, and at the end of the year, was elected to the Colonial Club, also carrying a managership. Colonial was one of the upper-class clubs where meals were served in the clubhouse. The duties of the manager were not strenuous. I had charge of the billiard room and the tobacco cabinet, and Bob Rinehard, the other manager, was in charge of the dining room. Also, at the end of the second year, I was offered a share in the managership of the Blakeley laundry, with Burt Hodgeman, then a junior and one of the best halfbacks on the varsity football team. This was a very busy job during the first two weeks of the opening of college, soliciting patrons for the laundry, and, in the middle and last part of the year, in collecting bills from the students who had used it. But this job more than paid my expenses and during my senior year it proved so lucrative that I saved enough money to pay my way through the first year in medical school.

At the end of my junior year I was visited by a man from Evanston, Illinois, who said that I had been recommended to him as a tutor for his son, a classmate of mine. He wanted me to spend the summer in Evanston tutoring his son in preparation for his re-examination in the fall. He said he would pay me $300 a month, and handed me a hundred-dollar bill for my traveling expenses. This offer, and a hundred-dollar bill which I had never seen before, was too good to refuse, for up to that time I had made no definite plans for the summer.

So I spent the summer in Evanston, with my mornings occupied in tutoring and evenings in studying the last six books of Virgil, which I had never read before, but which I had to teach my classmate. He was lazy, but bright, and he used to twit me, saying that I had to study harder than he to keep ahead of him. He was a very congenial fellow and we got along well. He introduced me to the game of golf, and coaching me among other things. I boarded in the home of a delightful family that had seen better days. Mrs. Lord set a very good table, and the fine meals with a select group of people made my stay there enjoyable. My afternoons were free, so that I spent a good many of them in nearby Chicago,

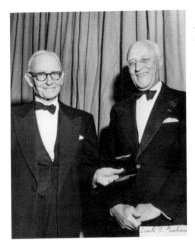

Dr Allen O. Whipple pictured here with Dr Evarts Graham.

attending the surgical clinics of Dr. David Graham, the father of my classmate, Evarts [6], also on the Princetonian Board. Dr. Graham was the Senior Surgeon at the Presbyterian Hospital, and Evarts was taking his first term in the Rush Medical School, so that I saw a good deal of him and his fine parents.

The senior year was by far the most interesting and enjoyable of my four years in Princeton. The work with "Spot" McClure [7] in biology was most stimulating. He had studied for two years at the College of Physicians and Surgeons, Columbia University, before he changed to biology as his lifework, and for many years had been associated with George S. Huntington [8], the famous anatomist in the College, in studying the development of the venous and lymphatic systems of the vertebrates. I had planned to attend the Johns Hopkins Medical School, but when McClure urged me to go to Columbia and said that he could get me a full scholarship there under Professor Huntington, I decided to study medicine in New York. Here again environment played a significant part in my life, for how different it would have been if I had gone to Baltimore. I am sure I would not have met my lovely Mary, and what a difference that would have made for the family and me! There were other courses that I enjoyed especially in my last two years at Princeton; one with Henry van Dyke on the English Lake poets; the other with Parrot (of course called "Polly"), in Shakespeare. Another was a seminar in Ethics under Francis Patton [9], who had been president of the university before Wilson took over in my junior year. Patton had one of the most brilliant minds that I ever encountered! He was lazy, but scintillating when he felt like it, and a born actor and mimic. If he had ever gone on the stage, he would have been another Jefferson. In the seminar, with only some twelve selected students, he revealed his real self to us.

In my junior year I had noticed that Enno Littmann offered an elective in Arabic. With my previous knowledge of the Syriac, a Semitic language much like the Arabic, I went to Littmann and asked him if he would accept me in his elective. He almost fell on me with joy, for he said no one had ever taken his elective before, and said he would accept me with pleasure. It was like having an expert tutor, for I was the only one in his class. It was held twice a week between two and three in the afternoon, but I frequently did not leave his library until five o'clock. If there was a question about the root of a word, in its Semitic connotations, he would climb his ladder to his bookshelves, and come down with three or four books and always get the answer. He was nearsighted and looked very much like the well-known picture of the bookworm with a book under each arm and between his legs. Because the faculty had a rule that an instructor could not flunk more than twenty percent of his class, my classmates unanimously elected me as the "class gut picker," a vulgar name for the man who picked the easiest course.

The work on the Princetonian during the last two years was not too strenuous, but interesting, and resulted in my coming to know not only the men in the classes, but many of the faculty members and the president. Woodrow Wilson [10] was an outstanding figure, a great speaker with an amazing command of English, and was a reformer of the university, which greatly needed it. He introduced the preceptorial system, which gave each group of ten to twenty students in a course the opportunity to meet one of the preceptors for an informal discussion of the topics that had been given in the lectures or in the required reading.

His choice of the first thirty preceptors was from top graduates of not only Princeton, but from universities all over the country. He also eliminated some of the dead wood in the faculty and introduced new courses that had been needed for a number of years. His work as president of the university will always go down in history as the most constructive and meaningful administration by any of its presidents.

The Monday Night Club was then an active organization, made up of some forty selected men from the two upper classes. They were chosen for their literary interests as well as their concern in public affairs. The Club met once a month to hear some prominent man in the country give an informal talk on his special interest or hobby. It was understood that there would be no report made of the talk given. I remember some of these sessions very clearly, especially when Colonel McClure, who had been one of the three secretaries of President Lincoln, the youngest of them and in many ways the one who came to know Lincoln most intimately during the most trying months of the Civil War, spoke to our group. He told us some of the most amusing stories that Lincoln had told him while he was waiting to see one of the many delegates that he insisted on seeing, and which took so much of his valuable time. He said the President used to come into McClure's office, off the reception room, sit in a long, low chair and put his feet high up on the mantle over the fireplace to "dreen my tired legs and feet." Most of the stories had never been published, for although they were seemingly funny and apt, they were not for the general public. Lincoln's rare sense of humor was often mixed with a barnyard and country store flavor as a result of his early days.

During senior year many of the class distinctions and rivalries disappeared, and a close class spirit helped us to evaluate then the lasting qualities of the men in the class. Senior singing on the steps of Nassau Hall, under the elms in the spring, was a delightful custom. For an hour after supper we would drift to the front campus and sit on the steps of the front door of Nassau Hall, to be led in singing old and new songs. The "faculty song", with verses caricaturizing members of the faculty, some kindly and others not, was always an amusing favorite.

Unfortunately this custom has faded out, for the movies and other distractions, which did not exist in our day, have eliminated the witching hour of former years, much to the distress of the older graduates. The disappearance of old customs is the result of larger classes and new distractions. In our time we lifted a senior through the window of the train when he left Princeton after graduating so that he could say that he never walked away from "the best place of all". In our senior year I was one of the last three to leave Princeton, so we took turns putting each other through the car windows. There is nothing left of that custom now.

From Princeton I returned to Duluth to find everyone well. The sisters had grown up, and Margaret and Mary were in High School; Eunice still in the grades. Lucius, who had roomed with me in Reunion Hall during my senior year, had decided to transfer to the University of Minnesota in Minneapolis. I had asked Evarts Graham to join me in a canoe trip through the Lake of the Woods country in Canada. We took a train north to the town of Ely on one of the lakes leading into Canada. There we bought our canoe, fishing gear and rifles, necessary for the trip, which we were taking without a guide, but with a compass and U.S. and Canadian district maps.

Ely was a primitive town and was the headquarters for the Indians who came from the north to sell their furs. We saw one family that had disposed of their pelts and were making queer use of their money. Two of the squaws had purchased and were wearing the most awful, gaudy hats, with red ostrich feathers rampant. The next day we passed this family in their canoe, the two squaws paddling, and the buck in the back of the canoe steering. The hats, gaudy no more, were resting on the bottom of the canoe with a dog sitting on one of them. As we paddled past the Indians, the buck asked us if we had any arnica; he said it was a good hot drink. He also asked us for the heel of our pipes; better he said, than chewing tobacco. If I had had much respect for the red man, I certainly lost it after seeing these and other Ojibwa Indians.

We had all the fish we could eat, as well as grouse that were so tame that we could knock them down with a stick. This was certainly wild

48

country that we were in. The only human beings we saw for ten days were a few Indians. But our enemy was the mosquito, unbelievably numerous, big, and vicious. Even a smudge in our tent and nets over our heads did not prevent their finding any vulnerable point, and they would drill through our blankets to find knees and elbows.

After we had been out ten days we left our canoe on the shore of the lake where we had camped and compassed our way to a smaller lake where the moose were said to be plentiful. We did not want to shoot them, but were after good photographs of them. Before we reached the smaller lake, some five miles from where we had left the canoe, we ran into a cloudburst that drenched us; then the hot sun appeared and dried us quickly. Evarts' new corduroy trousers promptly shrank so much that he had to cut the outside seams on either side so that he could climb over the windfalls that we had to cross. On our way back I discovered that our compass was behaving queerly, and from the position of the sun we knew we could not depend on it. Fortunately we had counted the ridges that we had crossed on our way in, so that after climbing the fifth one we came onto a lake that looked like the one we had left, but did not see any canoe. We agreed that one of us should walk east and the other west along the shore of the lake, and fire his rifle if he found the canoe. Evarts had not covered more than a quarter of a mile when I heard his gun. But it was after sundown and the mosquitoes were out in full force. They soon discovered the slits in Evarts' trousers and made him very miserable. We decided then and there to return to Ely, which we did without difficulty, for we knew the portages and the maps showed us the way without the need of a compass.

After Evarts had left Duluth, Lucius and I decided to work on the Iron Range north of Duluth. We had no difficulty in getting a job, which consisted in loading iron ore onto freight cars, and were paid on the basis of filling fifty-ton cars by wheeling the ore from the stockpiles in wheelbarrows. After four days of this backbreaking and hand-blistering work, we decided that we could do better by going out to the North Dakota wheat fields. So we took a harvester train, wearing our iron ore stained shirts and overalls, and rode to the end of one of the branches of the Northwestern Rail Road to an eleven-month-old town in North Dakota, named West Hope. On this night-train the majority of the men were miners, lumberjacks and day laborers. Knowing that they were going into a prohibition state, they had stocked up with flasks of whiskey. But these were soon emptied during the long night ride. Such a wild and drunken gang would be hard to find or describe. The conductor and brakeman put men off the train, many of them comatose, at the stations indicated by their tickets.

We arrived in West Hope in the late afternoon, registered at the only so-called hotel, a crude clapboard affair, and after dinner walked out to see the town. We came across a crowd of fellows engaged in putting the shot, in very clumsy fashion. Lucius, who had worked on the track team in high school and Princeton, was asked to take a try at it. He knew the technique and was in fine form. With his first heave, he put the shot eight feet further than any of the others. This gave him immediate recognition, and that evening we were offered four jobs, three of them after we had accepted one of digging a cellar for a new house.

After finishing this job, and after we had loaded a freight car with wheat bags, we were approached by a builder who asked if we could shingle roofs. This sounded much easier than the other jobs we had done, but we said we had no carpenter tools with us. He said he would furnish them. For the next two weeks we shingled the roof of the new church that was being built, the first one in the town. We then hired out to a wheat rancher who lived fifteen miles out of town on the prairie. He and his younger brother had taken a homestead claim of 640 acres before we arrived, and were raising hay, barley, and wheat. We found ourselves two of a group of six workers, two of them hoboes, one a Swede, another a jolly ex-convict who had recently been in jail for selling liquor to the Indians. We slept in the hay in the barn, and were awakened in the early morning by Lil Stair, the older of the brothers, pounding on the barn door with a baseball bat.

We had our meals with the farmer's family in their sod-roofed house. Lil Stair, formerly a mountaineer from West Virginia, could not make out who we were, but he said he was sure that "we had had some larnin". It was not cricket, in that time and country, to ask where a man came from - too many of them did not want it known! He could not remember my name, so he called me Sam, and gave me the job of milking his six cows. One of them had tried to jump a barbwire fence with dire results to her milk apparatus, and to me every time I had to milk her. To Lu he gave the job of feeding the pigs. Of course we had to do these chores, as well as watering and harnessing the horses, before going out to the fields. At six-thirty, after chores and breakfast, we started for the hay-fields where we worked until noon. By then the jugs of water were empty; they were warm by ten o'clock, and we learned as never before what a passion thirst could be. On our way back to the farmhouse we passed a patch of carrots, and ate four or five of them for their sugar and water content.

The two hoboes were hard workers, but no one, not even they knew when they would get the yen to move on, call for their pay and ride off on their bicycles. One of them did this only two weeks after we had arrived. The other had been a fireman on a freight engine, and had his union card with him. He said it was good at anytime, and he had used it crossing the continent more than once in his wanderings.

One of the old fellows that we met in the town of West Hope was called "Pop"; no one knew his name or asked it or where he was from. He spotted us for college men and on more than one occasion discussed Darwin, Spencer, and even quoted Jimmie McCosh [11], former beloved president of Princeton. He was obviously a very well educated man, but with a past that he did not want to disclose. One of the young fellows who had crossed into Canada, not more than fifteen miles from West Hope, returned intoxicated. He approached Pop while we were talking with him and made an insulting remark, at the same time grabbing the old man's arm. Like a flash Pop pulled out a long knife and said, "Touch me and you touch steel." The young fellow sobered in fast time and apologized to Pop.

We pitched hay for the first two weeks and then shocked wheat behind the reaper and binder, working from six-thirty till eight at night because of the threat of rust, a fungus that overnight could ruin a wheat farm. This fungus was blown from one area to another, all the way from Texas to the north. The sun seemed to stay in one spot from four o'clock until we left the fields, tired and consumed with thirst. But with all this hard work we gained weight, for our appetites were enormous and we had good food aplenty. For dessert each of us frequently had half a loaf of home-baked bread with plenty of butter and sorghum molasses.

Harvesting was over by the first of September, so we took a train for home, but at a fare three times the one we had paid on the harvester train, and because of our disreputable clothes and untrimmed beards, we weren't allowed on the Pulman car. But when we reached home, hot baths, sharp razors and regular clothes soon restored us to respectability.

Footnotes

1. **Laurence Hutton (1843-1904)**

   An American writer, a literary critic, a collector of death masks, and handwritten manuscripts, especially theatre-related. He is noted for a series of volumes describing literary pilgrimages in England, Italy, and many other lands.

2. **Enno Littmann (1875-1958)**

   A German researcher in "Oriental Studies". He took part in the first and the second American archaeological expedition in Syria and Palestine (1898-1900, 1904-1905) teaching at Princeton University in between. He became a Professor of Oriental Studies in Bonn from 1918 until his death in Tübingen.

3. **Edwin Booth (1833-1893)**

   An American actor. After years of touring with his father, Junius Brutus Booth, he appeared in New York City (1857) and later toured England (1861-63). On returning to New York he leased the Winter Garden Theatre, where in 1864 he presented his famous 100-night run of *Hamlet*. Booth endured the legacy left him by his brother - the assassin of Abraham Lincoln: his productions at the Winter Garden terminated in 1865, when his brother John Wilkes Booth assassinated the President. The ensuing scandal forced Booth to retire, but he returned to the Winter Garden in 1866. When it burned down, he built Booth's Theatre, New York (1869).

4. **John McCullough (1837-1885)**

    Born in Ireland, he came to America at the age of sixteen, and made his first appearance on the stage at the Arch Street Theatre, Philadelphia, in 1857. In support of Edwin Forrest and Edwin Booth he played second roles in Shakespearian and other tragedies. His life was tragically ended when he was arguing with another actor over a coveted role in one of the performances; the less reputable actor shot and killed McCullough in the backstage area. The theatre claims that McCullough's ghost haunts the premises ever since.

5. **Joseph Jefferson (1829-1905)**

    Considered as one of the most popular comic actors in America through the end of the 19th century. Jefferson achieved his first great success in 1858 in Tom Taylor's *Our American Cousin*. He is best remembered for his portrayal in the 1860s of *Rip Van Winkle*, an Americanized version of a German folk tale popularized by Washington Irving in *The Sketch Book of Geoffrey Crayon, Gent* (1819-1820). Americans loved his portrayal of *Rip Van Winkle* so much that Jefferson never created another role for himself.

6. **Evarts Graham (1883-1957)**

    Chairman of the Department of Surgery at Washington University School of Medicine and Surgeon-in-Chief at Barnes Hospital from 1919 to 1951. He performed the first successful pneumonectomy for cancer in 1933 and introduced cholecystography to evaluate the biliary tree. He, along with his first year medical student, Ernst Wynder (1922-1999) reported *Tobacco smoking as a possible etiological factor in bronchogenic carcinoma* in the *Journal of the American Medical Association* (1950). He was a co-founder of the American Board of Surgery. More than 40 of his trainees went on to become department chairmen or heads of specialty services, a tribute to his focus on surgical education and training.

7. **Charles McClure (1865-1955)**

    Professor of Biology at Princeton University. Among other things, he collected some 1200 letters sent to him by some 400 biologists and anatomists of the academic community in the United States and throughout the world. In his assay, *The*

Monastery, McClure described the living arrangements of various groups of junior faculty at Princeton from the 1880s until 1937.

8. **George Huntington (1861-1925)**

Although a surgeon by training, he was Columbia's and the nation's first Professor of Anatomy, who revolutionized the study of anatomy in US medical schools. Before Huntington, medical students learned anatomy by sitting at the feet of lecturers who hurried through their work in order to devote the chief part of their time to surgery. Huntington introduced the laboratory method of teaching human anatomy. He once said: "Anatomy is not an offshoot of surgery but is a science of itself and should be regarded and taught as such". Huntington's collection of anatomical material, perhaps the largest collection in the world, included some 5,000 specimens, illustrating the form, development, and evolution of most parts of the body in many species, including man. These comparative specimens are currently at the Smithsonian Institution's Museum of Natural History, 10th Street and Constitution Ave., NW, Washington, D.C. 20560. Huntington should not be confused with George Sumner Huntington (1850-1916) for whom Huntington's chorea is named.

9. **Francis Landey Patton (1843-1932)**

The 12th president of Princeton University. During his administration, Princeton's student body increased from slightly over 600 to more than 1300, and the faculty doubled. Faculty accounts indicate that Patton lacked initiative in important policy matters, resisted meaningful curriculum reform, was lax in matters of discipline and in scholarly standards. As one faculty member put it, he was "a wonderfully poor administrator". He was succeeded by Woodrow Wilson.

10. **Woodrow Wilson (1856-1924)**

Nicknamed the "schoolmaster in politics" he is chiefly remembered for his high-minded idealism, which appeared both in his leadership on the faculty and in the presidency of Princeton University (1902-1910), and in his national and world statesmanship during and after World War I (1913-1921). A Nobel laureate for peace (1919) and the only US President to hold a Ph.D. degree.

11. **James McCosh (1811-1894)**

A Scottish writer who became a minister of the Church of Scotland and later took part in the Free Church movement. In 1852 he was appointed Professor of Logic and Metaphysics in Queen's College, Belfast and in 1868 was chosen President and Professor of Philosophy at Princeton, New Jersey.

Chapter Six

Medical School

1904 - 1908

The next week saw me in New York to begin work in the College of Physicians and Surgeons on 59th Street. Three of my classmates in Princeton were in the first year class: Arch Strong, with whom I roomed, Wesley Bowers [1] and Frank Sloane. We soon met two very attractive Yale men, Gene Soper and Tony Waring, both bones men. The six of us were appointed as prosectors in anatomy to the two instructors in that subject. This gave us special training in that subject, for we had to make demonstration dissections for the instructors to be shown to the class. Strong, Bowers and I boarded and roomed at 345 West 58th Street, about two blocks from the medical school. The landlady was a southerner and a very good cook, whose only interest was her yellow cat, Nosey. Her husband was a Harvard Law graduate, able and indispensable to the Sheriff's office. But he was a dipsomaniac, and periodically Mrs. Lincoln would ask one of us to bring him home from the corner saloon, which he always patronized. He was never angry or mean when we urged him to come home, and thanked us through his clicking dentures. The rest of the company at the boarding house and the dining table was the weirdest mixture of people imaginable. In fact we said that the current play, *The Third Floor Back*, must have been based on this apartment and company. There was an actor and his wife, a Spanish riding master, one of the lewdest reprobates to be found anywhere, a French porcelain agent from Limoge, and two ladies of uncertain age and occupation. Probably the only thing that preserved our morals in that bawdy neighborhood was the fact that we were very busy in our studies and had to keep our noses close to the grindstone.

Our class in the medical school was very different from the one in Princeton, made up of some 160 men of different ages and nationalities; there were no women in the school at that time. The oldest student was a brother of General Pershing [2], forty-seven years old and not brilliant; the youngest, eighteen, was very bright. In later years he became the senior medical attending at the Mt. Sinai Hospital and the President of the New York Academy of Medicine. We had some able professors, George S. Huntington, a worldwide figure in comparative and human anatomy, as was T. M. Prudden [3] in pathology. I came to know two of the young instructors especially well. Bill Darrach [4], who later was Dean of the Medical School, and Bill Clarke [5], a surgical pathologist. I worked with both of these rare characters for twenty-five years in the surgical department.

Bill Clarke was a very unusual fellow, a keen observer and a born naturalist and ornithologist although he was color-blind. As a teacher he was a peripatetic, and Socratic in his methods. I never saw him sit at his desk in the course he gave in first year surgery. He read little and published less. In quizzing his class, if one of them quoted an authority or text, Bill would say, "How do you know that is so?" He said this so frequently that he soon was called "How do you know Clarke," and a good many of the class never did. I was in the first class that he taught. Several years later when he started to write a textbook on the *Fundamentals of Surgery* he became so involved in making sure that his statements were true and that the words he was using gave the exact meaning that he wanted, that he never finished the book and was still revising the first chapter. I worked in his laboratory three summers and got a fine background of surgical pathology with him. I also came to know him as one of my closest friends and associates in the surgical department.

Huntington was a master in comparative anatomy. He was very handsome with a deep bass voice and gave wonderful lectures, which were frequently over the heads of most of the second year class. He told me once that he was really only interested in the top ten men in the class, and complemented me by appointing me as his head prosector in my second year, always considered a top honor. This gave me further experience in anatomy and the privilege of working with Huntington and the other instructors in his department.

Besides the course in surgery with Bill Clarke, we had bacteriology with Zinsser [6], medicine with Evans [7] and pathology with Prudden. Clarke, Zinsser and Evans were stimulating teachers whom I came to know well in later years. During the summer that I worked with Clarke in his laboratory at the College, I had as a running mate a classmate, Ben Michaelovsky. He was older than I and had been educated at Russian and German universities. Like so many Russians, he was brilliant and ready to argue on every subject. We had many discussions and pleasant trips on the Staten Island ferry, which we found to be the greatest relief after the broiling summer days on 59th Street.

In my third year a group of us: St. John, West, Tooker, McAlpin, Philips and Bowers (all Princeton men), Burnap, Eli, and Johnson (a Williams's graduate), rented a house on west 65th Street. We took our meals at Childs' restaurant or the nearby Empire Hotel. We were a congenial and hard-working group and came to know each other well, with all the individualities and idiosyncrasies of the different fellows that were in different classes in the medical school.

I had two jobs in the school that helped pay my expenses: one was to be in charge of the Bone Room where human bones, in set boxes, were distributed to the first year students for their course in anatomy; the other job was that of night librarian. This kept me in the library from 7 to 9:30 five nights a week, but it gave me fairly uninterrupted study hours with plenty of books and magazines for reference.

At the end of our third year I was recommended by Gene Soper to the Jennings family in Bennington, Vermont, as tutor for their son, Fritz. They owned a large farm and beautiful home north of Mt. Anthony; it was later given to found the Bennington College for Women. Their large house on Park Avenue in New York was, years later, purchased by the Princeton Club of that city. Mr. Jennings was one of the leading corporation lawyers in New York. He was a man of character with the kindest of dispositions, but with an austere manner.

My duties that summer were anything but strenuous. They consisted of playing tennis and golf, and riding horseback with fourteen-year old Fritz and his seventeen-year old sister, Elsie. They had many guests, including one crowd of boys of Fritz' age that I had to take on a camping trip and act as cook. Their appetites were amazing, but I found that by filling them with oatmeal was the best way of keeping them satisfied during the morning. Swimming and fishing were the chief occupations during the ten-day trip.

I was glad to get back to New York and the beginning of the last year in medical school. The climax and end of all of the courses at that time were the hospital appointments to internships. Preparing for them started from the day we entered the school. Although I had been Huntington's head prosector in my second year, and Blake's during my last two years, I was very worried about the prospects of getting an internship at the Roosevelt Hospital, where I was eager to serve under Blake [8], the Professor of Surgery at Columbia. He and Brewer [9] were the two senior surgeons at the Roosevelt. I felt that I was especially handicapped because I had to pass up the examinations for the Presbyterian and St. Luke's Hospitals that came before the ones at the Roosevelt. As a result of this worry I went into a mild depression during the fall of the last year, along with others in the class. We called ourselves the manic depressives.

Two days before Christmas, while I was on the out-patient obstetrical service, I delivered an Irish woman in the Hell's Kitchen district. She and her husband were drunk and would have nothing to do with the newborn infant. My efforts to keep it alive on formula milk were not successful, and on Christmas Eve it breathed its last. When I announced the fact to the parents, all the father did was to tell me to call the undertaker. I returned to my room in the out-patient department opposite the Roosevelt Hospital, tired and depressed after my experience with the Irish parents. When I reached my room I found that Johnnie St. John had sent me a copy of Dickens' Christmas Carol. I had never read it, but when I started it that evening I did not put it down until I had finished it. It was like a tonic and I felt made over, went to bed and slept soundly.

During the night it had snowed hard and the Christmas morning was very like the one described in the last few pages of the Carol. I suddenly felt cheerful and confident as I waved to Dick Derby across the street in the Roosevelt Hospital. Then and there I decided to burn my bridges and prepare for the Roosevelt examination and Blake's service. From then on I was able to apply myself consistently, and by April, when the examinations were held, I was appointed to the Roosevelt and got Blake's service. At the end of the year I tied for third place in the final rating.

Footnotes

1. **Wesley C. Bowers (-1963)**
    A graduate of the P & S of Columbia in 1908. He held a position in the department of surgery between 1924 until 1944 becoming an assistant clinical Professor of Surgery in 1940.

2. **John Joseph Pershing (1860-1948)**
    Commander-in-Chief of the American Expeditionary Forces in WWI, and the General of the Armies of the United States (one rank above five-star general) by a special act of the congress. Winner of the Pulitzer Prize for history (1932) for his memoirs *My Experience in the World War.*

3. **Theophil M. Prudden (1849-1924)**
    A physician, pathologist, bacteriologist, and a central figure in the scientific medical life of New York. After graduating form Yale Medical School he went to Europe to work under Julius Arnold, Rudolf Virchow, Robert Koch, and F.A.T Hueppe. He was the first to make diphtheria antitoxin in the United States, used to check an epidemic of diphtheria in New York City.

4. William Darrach (1876-1948)

The Head of the P & S Surgical Division at Bellevue Hospital, and the Dean of the College from 1919.

5. William Coggswell Clarke (-1943)

Joined the faculty of the P & S of Columbia University in 1901 and became a Professor of Experimental Surgery in 1926.

6. Hans Zinsser (1878-1940)

A physician, bacteriologist and author who collaborated with Dr. Philip H. Hiss, Jr., in a series of papers and in the first edition of the *Textbook of Bacteriology* (1910). The last 17 years of his life he spent at Harvard University Medical School as Professor of Bacteriology and Immunology and an expert on typhoid fever.

7. Evan M. Evans (1870-1955)

Professor of Clinical Medicine at the P & S of Columbia University from 1909 to 1938, who was known as a "unique diagnostician".

8. Joseph A. Blake (1864-1937)

Professor of Surgery and the Head of Department of Surgery at P & S of Columbia University. (1903-1913). Just prior to WWI he resigned his position and went to Europe. During the war he offered his services to France, where he gained charge of six American military hospitals in Paris, winning a rank of Colonel. He is best known for the "Blake Splint" for leg fractures.

9. George Emerson Brewer (1861-1939)

A Professor of Clinical Surgery at P & S of Columbia University and attending surgeon at the Roosevelt and Presbyterian Hospitals. During WWI he served in France; here he was a member of the surgical team that tried to save Edward Revere Osler (1895-1917), Sir William Osler's only son, who was injured in a battlefield.

Chapter Seven

Roosevelt Hospital - Internship

1909 - 1911

My two years' surgical internship at the hospital did not begin until the following January 1909, so that I had six months of free time. Dr. George Brewer asked me to ride herd on his two boys during the summer. This again was more or less a sinecure job, for the boys 10 and 7 years old did not have to be tutored. The first part of the summer was spent in Southampton, on Long Island, where we did not have much to do except to play tennis and swim in the ocean. Mrs. Brewer was a delightful woman, with a fine sense of humor that came to the rescue in many of the contacts with the foreign diplomatic corps that made their headquarters in that town during the summer. I got to know a Harvard graduate about my age and with a similar occupation. We became surf devotees and frequently went in when the waves were too high for the rest of the crowd. It was amusing to watch the foreign diplomats at the strict society hour of 11 to 12 disporting themselves not too far in the ocean. I remember seeing one lady wearing silk stockings and high-heeled slippers. She did not venture above her covered knees; a Frenchman sporting a straw hat and a monocle did not do more than sit in the shallow surf.

In August we went to the Adirondacks to the Tahaus Club, where Mrs. Brewer and the boys, expert with rod and fly, caught many a speckled trout in the lakes and streams of the club preserves. Having had some experience in the streams on the north shore of Lake Superior, I did my

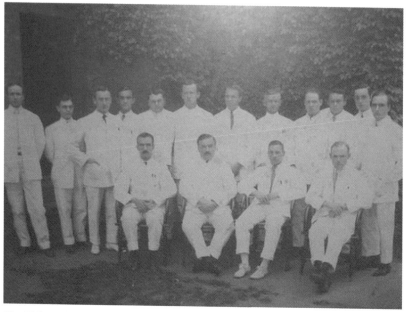

Dr Whipple (third from left) with the house staff at The Roosevelt Hospital.

share of catching the trout. The trails through the woods were well blazed, so the hikes were many and safe as were the mountain climbs.

On January 1, 1909, I began my surgical internship at the Roosevelt. My duties in the first six months were to give the anesthesia in the operating room in the morning, with laboratory work and taking histories and doing physical examinations in the afternoon. I had had no experience in giving anesthesia, an art that I had to learn by experience, at my expense as well as that of some of the patients during the first month. But I found that I could give a better anesthetic by the open drop ether method than with the Bennett apparatus, and during the six months as a junior I gave over 600 such anesthesias. We had an ambulance service and an active emergency ward, so there were many emergency operations on our receiving nights, three times a week.

I worked with Richard Derby [1], a delightful Harvard graduate, who married Ethel Roosevelt, the daughter of Theodore Roosevelt. He later settled in Oyster Bay, the leading surgeon on Long Island. Another man on the team was Bill Ward, a Mormon from Utah. He had taken the July appointment and was the second senior when I was his junior. He later settled in Salt Lake City and became the leading surgeon there.

Joseph A. Blake was the senior surgeon, Walton Martin [2], the associate, and Adrian Lambert [3] and Karl Connell [4] the juniors on the second surgical division. Blake was a master surgeon, a surgeon's surgeon. As a great anatomist, his sharp knife dissections at the operating table were clean, finished and models for all of us younger men. He had the best surgical judgment of any man that I ever knew. As Professor of Surgery at the College he was greatly admired and had a very select practice. He was his own most severe critic, and when he criticized the work of others or corrected their mistakes it was always deserved, and he never held a grudge against anyone, but was the first to praise another's accomplishments.

Martin was a scholar, not only in surgery, but also in other medical fields. He was an omnivorous reader and had a wide knowledge of world literature. A bachelor, he had traveled abroad extensively, especially in Italy, and knew the language and lore of that country. He later was appointed Chief of Surgery at St. Luke's Hospital and married a wealthy widow. In later years he became known as the surgical philosopher because of the sound and finished articles that he contributed to the surgical literature.

Lambert had overcome the handicap of the loss of an eye, the result of an infection that occurred while he was operating as a house surgeon at the New York hospital. He was one of three brother doctors prominent in New York. His oldest brother, Sam, was, for a number of years, the dean of the medical school, and while I was a medical student there. Adrian was also a scholar and an able surgeon. He had a great sense of humor, with one of the most robust laughs. But he had an equally hot temper, which got the better of him at times when it compromised his better judgment and his operative skill.

Connell was more of a gadgeteer than a surgeon. He developed a fine apparatus for giving anesthesia, and his inventive bent was again shown during the First World War in developing the gas mask that was used in the army. Like so many men of his type, he did not have the shred of a sense of humor and was not easy to work with.

During my second six months I was second senior on the medical service. Evan Evans [5] was the senior physician, a brilliant diagnostician and a born teacher. A profound student, familiar with medical literature, he never published anything, saying that too much trash had already been published. Like Bill Clarke, whom he knew well, he was color-blind and an ornithologist, but unlike Bill, he was a musician and played the piano well. Bill said that singing made him feel like howling.

Evans' associate, whose name I have fortunately forgotten, was a fat, lazy fellow, in charge of the service during the summer. As interns we had no respect for him. That summer and fall we had a severe epidemic of typhoid fever, which kept doctors and nurses busy day and night. I helped take care of 96 such patients, and the women's ward was given up entirely to the typhoid cases. At that time the accepted treatment was to tub the patients every four hours, for those who had temperatures over 101 degrees, in water at 65 degrees. It was a cruel routine, exhausting to the patients, as well as to the nurses, doctors and orderlies. Since then this treatment has been entirely replaced with rational dietary and intravenous fluid therapy.

This incidence of typhoid during the summer and fall probably had much to do with the presence of flies and uncovered fruit and food supplies in the open markets. At the present time typhoid has almost disappeared in our cities due to typhoid inoculations, maintaining pure water and milk supplies, and removing gall bladders from typhoid carriers. During my surgical service at the Presbyterian Hospital I had the opportunity of operating upon 32 carriers, an example of preventive surgery.

During that summer a very significant thing happened which took the leading role at Physicians and Surgeons of Columbia from the Roosevelt Hospital and gave it to the Presbyterian Hospital. Edward Harkness [6], one of the greatest philanthropists in this country, had been especially interested in medical education, through some of his classmates at Yale who were the leading physicians in and out of New York, especially Bill Darrach. He offered a sum of several million dollars to Columbia University and the Roosevelt Hospital if they would unite to organize a University Hospital. The president of the Board of Trustees of the Roosevelt at that time was James McLane [7], a stubborn Scot who had been dean of the medical school. He had become involved in a bitter controversy with President Butler of Columbia over basic policies in the conduct of the medical school, which resulted in his forced resignation. McLane who had a vote on the hospital board and a permanent grudge against Columbia, cast the deciding vote against accepting the offer that Harkness had made, a decision that set the hospital back for many years.

Harkness turned to the Presbyterian and its board accepted the offer, as did Columbia. This meant a reorganization of the Presbyterian staff. Blake resigned from the surgical service of the Roosevelt, and went to the Presbyterian to organize the teaching program in the new University Hospital. Blake took with him Lambert, Clarke and Auchincloss [8], which was a sad blow to those of us on the intern staff of the Roosevelt who had wanted to complete their training under Blake and his associates.

However, Charles Peck [9], the associate with Brewer on the first surgical division, was appointed to be the senior surgeon on the second division to succeed Blake. This was a happy choice, for Peck was considered one of the ablest of the young surgeons in the city, and pleased all of us on the second division as a compensation for the loss of our idol, Blake. Peck was modest, with impeccable character, and a great man to work with. I shall always consider my training with him on a par with what I had had with Blake, Martin and Lambert.

During my six months as house surgeon under Peck, I was given more than my share of operative work. In fact, I gained in his estimation when

I asked him to let me assist him in some of the cases that he had turned over to me, because I said that I was sure that it would be to the patients' advantage if he would operate. One of the associate surgeons had the bad habit of turning over bad risk patients with little chance of recovery so that he would not increase his mortality rate.

This was before the days of residency training in New York. Halsted [10] had started the long-term residency program in the Johns Hopkins Hospital fifteen years before, but few other clinics in America had adopted his program of appointing residents after their internship training. The New York hospitals had a strong prejudice against Halsted because of the change in him and his surgery, following his tragic experience in New York where he innocently acquired the cocaine habit, against which he had made such a soul-trying fight. The physical and mental effort to overcome the habit had changed him from a brilliant, rapid operator to a slow, meticulous surgeon, and from an extrovert to a shy, reserved introvert. But his experience of more than one year in the Butler Hospital in Providence, Rhode Island, had given him time to develop the surgical philosophy that resulted in his establishing the great school of surgery in Baltimore that is now recognized all over the world.

In the New York hospitals when I was house surgeon, the surgical interns with periods of 18 to 24 months of training, took all the operative work given them. When they left they worked in the out-patient departments of the hospitals with no further operative experience. The only surgery they did was at the expense of what private patients they could get. Many of them went into general practice and did no further surgery; their surgical training was entirely wasted.

Before I began my work at the Presbyterian I had accepted an appointment as a summer resident at the Sloane Hospital for Women, to work in obstetrics. There I learned the folly of fixed routine, for the Sloane Hospital had it in the worst form. Certain things had to be done to the patients regardless of how large or how small, how heavy or thin. If a small, thin woman lost nineteen ounces of blood during her delivery, nothing was said about it in the doctor's record. But if a large, two hundred and fifty pounder lost twenty ounces, one had to fill out an elaborate sheet that was worse than making out an income tax return. Every patient in the wards was given five grains of calomel at night, regardless of her need for it, or her size. This certainly kept the nurses busy with the bedpans.

I was unpopular with the head of the nursing school because one night, as the senior resident, I had to deliver fourteen women. This used up all the sterile supplies in the place. In reply to the caustic remarks of the dowager, I insisted that it was not my fault if all fourteen of the patients decided to go into labor the same night.

Footnotes

1. **Richard Derby (1881-1963)**
    Son-in-law of President Theodore Roosevelt. At the outset of WWI he was a surgeon at the American Ambulance Hospital in Paris. He served as a division surgeon receiving the Croix de Guerre and the French Legion of Honor, and the Distinguished Service Medal.

2. **Walton Martin (-1949)**
    On the faculty of P & S of Columbia University from 1897, he became a Professor of Clinical Surgery in 1913 until 1947. He served as a consultant at St. Luke's Hospital and was among those who treated Theodore Roosevelt and Nicolas Murray Butler. He is an author of many books and articles in surgery, including the revision of *Green's Pathology*. During WWI he served at the American Hospital in Paris.

3. **Adrian Van S. Lambert (1872-1952)**
    A member of the faculty of the P & S of Columbia University for 45 years, and the brother of Samuel Lambert, Dean of the P & S (1904-1919). He founded and directed the thoracic surgery service. In 1907 he was credited with successfully directing the first transfusion for hemorrhagic disease of the newborn (his own newborn daughter). He was a co-founder of the American Board of Surgery.

4. Carl A. Connell (-1941)

A faculty member of the P & S of Columbia University who invented an anesthetic apparatus. As a major in the US Army Medical Corps during WWI he received the Distinguished Service Medal.

5. Evan M. Evans (1870-1955)

Professor of Clinical Medicine at the P & S of Columbia University from 1909 to1938 who was known as a "unique diagnostician".

6. Edward S. Harkness (1874-1940)

A philanthropist interested in the prevention and cure of disease. Harkness' gifts to humanity totaled more than $130,000,000. Once, holding a dollar, he said: "A dollar misspent is a dollar lost and we must not forget that some man's work made this dollar." But another time, when a friend was urging caution in some extensive philanthropy, he said with a twinkle: "What's the use of having money if you can't have the fun of spending it?"

7. James McLane (1839-1912)

An obstetrician and the first director of the Sloane Maternity Hospital (NY) and President of the Vanderbilt Clinic (NY). He designed and used the McLane forceps for many years before mentioning them in his 1981 account of the first 1,000 deliveries at Sloane Hospital. In 1889 he became the President of P & S. As personal physician to the Vanderbilts he had influence over the direction of his patients' philanthropy and thus responsible for the enormous benefits accrued to P & S through the Vanderbilts' generosity.

8. Hugh Auchincloss (1878-1947)

A graduate of the P & S of Columbia University in 1905 who founded the surgical pathology laboratory. During the 1918 influenza epidemic he developed the "Auchincloss tube" for drainage of the pleural cavity. In 1932 he presented his collection of more than 300 autograph letters, pictures and other souvenirs of Florence Nightingale to the Columbia-Presbyterian Medical Center School of Medicine.

9. **Charles H. Peck (1870-1927)**

A graduate of P & S of Columbia University in 1892, a senior surgeon and a Professor of Surgery since 1910. During WWI in France, he organized a 3,000-bed hospital at the Chaumont. He was awarded the Distinguished Service Medal, made an honorary member of the 68th Alpine Chasseurs of the French Army, and an officer of L'instruction Publique. He was the President of the American Surgical Association, and a member of board of reagents for the American College of Surgeons. He died of pernicious anemia.

10. **William Stewart Halsted (1852-1922)**

As the first Professor of Surgery at the Johns Hopkins Hospital, Halsted has left an indelible mark on American surgery to the present day. Halsted's greatest contribution was the residency system for training surgeons. His aim was to train surgical teachers, not merely competent operating surgeons. Halsted introduced a "new" American surgery, based on pathology, physiology, as well as on anatomy. His list of accomplishments includes: pioneering the use of cocaine for local anesthesia (he himself abused cocaine) and introducing a host of surgical techniques for dealing with cancers, goiters, hernias, and aneurysms. During his three decades of chairmanship, seven of his chief residents became full professors of surgery at other universities, including: Harvey Cushing (1869-1939) at Harvard University; Stephen Watts (1877-1953) at the University of Virginia; George Heuer (1882-1950) at the Universities of Cincinnati and Cornell, NY; Mont Reid (1889-1943) at the University of Cincinnati; John Churchman (1877-1937) at Yale University; Robert Miller (1886-1960) at the University of Pittsburgh; and Emile Holman (1890-1977) at Stanford University. In addition, Roy McClure (1882-1951) was named Surgeon-in-Chief at the Henry Ford Hospital, Detroit, and James Mitchell (1871-1961) became Professor of Clinical Surgery at George Washington University.

Chapter Eight

The Presbyterian Hospital

1911 - 1915

On January 1st, 1911, I began work at the Presbyterian under Blake, Lambert, Clarke and Auchincloss. They made up the attending staff of the new teaching surgical service. The Presbyterian at that time was on 70th Street, between Madison and Park Avenues. Small in comparison with the present Medical Center, it had the reputation of being conservative and, in the eyes of its competitors, self satisfied and smug. Certainly this was true to a certain extent, especially with regard to men like the austere Superintendent, Dr. Irving Fisher [1]. When I entered the hospital on the first morning on duty, I was told that the doctor wished to see me. When I entered his office he said, "Doctor, I understand that you have been having your mail forwarded to this hospital. I hope that you are not doing this for advertising purposes." I said, "Doctor Fisher, that never occurred to me, but it is not a bad idea." He had no sense of humor, so that my remark only made him suspicious of me.

Miss Anna Maxwell [2] was the supervisor of nurses, one of the outstanding women in that field. She was a grand dame, one whom we all admired and respected. She was a martinet with the nurses, but with a heart, and she had developed one of the best, if not the best, training schools for nurses in the country.

Having the medical students in the hospital wards as clinical clerks on both the medical and surgical services changed the entire tone of the place to that of a university center. It did away with the moss-grown conservative attitude that had previously existed. The laboratory space was greatly enlarged and research was given first place in the program. Theodore Janeway [3] was appointed to the Chair of Medicine, and Will MacCallum [4] to the Chair of Pathology. My work at first was directing the work of the clinical clerks in the morning, with work in the surgical laboratory from one to three o'clock, then across town to the laboratory at P & S on 59th street. There John MacWhorter [5] and I were studying the development of the earliest blood vessels in the chick embryo. After incubating the eggs for 48 hours in a regular incubator, we removed the embryo in the so-called blastoderm stage and transferred it to a hanging drop of chicken plasma. This we placed on a glass slide and put the slide on the stage of a microscope. This microscope was housed in a small incubator, kept at a constant temperature of 38 degrees Centigrade. The eyepiece of the microscope projected above the top of the incubator, and the screw adjustment to the right side of the same. This made it possible to study the growth of the embryo and take photomicrographs at desired intervals. In this way we were able to observe the first blood islands, the rotation of the four chambers of the heart, and to see the first heartbeat starting the circulation of the blood. The small space of the hanging drop and the limited supply of nourishing plasma prevented our observing this development beyond the 70 to 90 hour period.

Our source of plasma supply was from the blood of an old rooster in the laboratory. He required a short ether anesthesia every time we tapped one of his veins. During the 14th donation he was given an overdose of ether, which ended the rooster's daily crowing. The Scotch doctor, who was responsible for the anesthesia death, took the remains home for a stew. He later acknowledged that the bird was a bit tough, and very bad tasting.

Much of our work with the embryos had to be done at night, for if we had a good specimen and were getting photographs every hour, we were sometimes in the laboratory all night and frequently did not leave until two in the morning. Mrs. MacWhorter was very tolerant but I am sure she blamed me, the bachelor of the team, for keeping her husband up to such late hours. They had been married for several years, but that spring they were expecting the first arrival. One morning about two o'clock, shortly before the child was born, I noticed that Mac was looking tired and worried. When I asked him what was the trouble, he said, "This business of having a baby is hell on the woman, but God only knows what it is for the man." The baby boy arrived four days later; he is now a practicing physician in Englewood.

Later that year at the December meeting of the American Association of Anatomists in Princeton, Huntington and McClure invited us to present the work we had been doing with the chick embryos before the Association, and sponsored our paper on *The Angiogenesis in the Living Embryo of the Chick*. At that time there was a rather acrid controversy between the Columbia - Princeton anatomists and the Johns Hopkins group over the origin of the blood and lymphatic vessels. Our studies favored the view of the former group. It is interesting that my first piece of research, and the last that I did in the Biology Laboratory in Princeton had to do with the circulation of the blood in the living animal.

During the first eighteen months after beginning my work at the Presbyterian I roomed with Ned Park [6] who was then working with Janeway on the effect of adrenalin on the smooth muscle of the guinea pig. We had an apartment at 981 Madison Avenue, and shared offices with Hugh Auchincloss, a very close friend to both of us. We first took our meals with the Auchincloss family who lived several floors above us, but after a few months Ned and I decided it would be wiser to hire a cook and have our meals in our own apartment. This would have worked well if we had managed to get a good cook. The one we engaged was a rather frail old woman, who knew very little of the art and was such a pathetic soul that neither Ned nor I had the heart to let her go.

Ned Park is one of the most interesting and delightful characters that I have ever known. Our friendship has continued over the years, increasing with time although we have been working in different cities ever since 1912. His sense of humor is one of the most subtle and delightful of his many sterling qualities. The stories of his absent-mindedness, and of the pranks that were played on his staff and that they played on him, should be recorded in a special volume to be distributed to his host of friends in the three universities where he worked as Professor of Pediatrics: Columbia, Yale and Johns Hopkins.

Two examples of his whimsies follow. The Park family lived in the picturesque house in Garrison when he was at the Johns Hopkins. Ned used to ride to and from the hospital on his old bicycle. Before he left home, Agnes, his wife, would slip a message to his secretary into Ned's coat pocket. When he arrived at the hospital and had changed to his long white coat, his secretary would take out the note and answer it, placing the note in Ned's regular coat. Agnes would recover this when Ned returned home. This went on for four or five years without his knowing about it. Agnes had found that Ned's absent-mindedness too often failed to relay her messages.

In 1921, after I had been appointed to the Chair of Surgery at Columbia, I went to Baltimore to consult with Dr. Halsted about matters connected with the organization of the department. Ned had arranged for this appointment to see the "Professor", as he was always called, at his home in the evening. This I heard later was a rare privilege, for very few people had ever had that opportunity. Ned met me at the Baltimore railroad station, where we had dinner before going to the Halsted home.

As we sat at dinner I saw him running his fingers through his hair, a gesture that I knew well, indicating that he had something amusing to tell. So I said, "Tell me about it." "Well," he said, "Yesterday morning after a heavy snowfall, I was walking toward the hospital, when I saw one of my residents walking a little ahead of me on the other side of the street. I reached down and made a snowball out of the wet snow and heaved it at him. He must have seen me for he ducked and the snowball crashed through the front window of the house opposite him. He waved his hand at me with a wicked grin and walked on. Of course I had to cross the street, ring the doorbell of the house where the damage had been done. A dear old lady opened the door and I announced myself as the culprit, and said that I wanted to pay for the window that I had broken. She said it was good of me to acknowledge the accident and told me the cost of the large windowpane. I reached for my wallet and discovered that in changing my suit that morning I had forgotten my money. Very embarrassed, I told her my predicament and said that I would call this morning. This I did, making sure of my wallet. When I rang the bell, a gentleman appeared and I announced that I had come to pay for the windowpane I had broken. He said, 'I am sorry, but I can't take your money.' After repeated refusals to accept the agreed sum, I said, 'Will you please tell me why you won't accept this money?' 'Well, if you insist on knowing, I have to tell you that the window you broke is next door!'"

In the spring of 1911 I was working in the laboratory at the college in the early afternoon when I was called to the phone to hear Arch Strong's voice. He said, "I want you to come to the Belmont Hotel to meet two young ladies from Woods Hole this afternoon at five." I said, "Arch, I am in the middle of an experiment that I can't leave, so you had better count me out and get someone else to help you do the honors." His reply was, "Oldfather, I am not in the habit of insisting that my invitation be accepted, but I am making an exception this time. You come to the Belmont without fail." So I could not say no, for I knew that Arch was very discriminating when it came to the ladies. I obeyed the summons. I went, I saw and was conquered. In the foyer of the hotel I first met Mary Neales and her sister, Margaret. If it were not love at first sight, it was because I did not dare it to be. But two more meetings, one at the Hippodrome with no recollection of the stage or the performance, made me realize that something new in my life, something that I would have to watch very carefully, had suddenly occurred, for here I was having very recently finished my hospital training and just beginning to practice with very little, if any, of the goods of this world.

Miss Neales - we did not call each other by first names as soon then as is done at present - had come to New York to arrange to have her sister admitted to the Nurses Training School at the Presbyterian Hospital. When this was accomplished, Miss Mary and Miss Margaret returned to Boston. I was careful to get her address, and during that summer there was an exchange of letters. After I had finished my residency at the Sloane Hospital I went to Boston, ostensibly on my way to Martha's Vineyard to visit the Auchinclosses and Ned Park. But I stopped at the Carney Hospital to call on Miss Neales who was recovering from an appendix operation. This led from one thing to another.

Later in the fall, when she was on her way to Thomasville with Miss Fay, we met in New York and had a memorable dinner on the roof of the Astor Hotel. She looked more charming and lovely, wearing a broad-brimmed straw hat, of a watermelon pink color. Our correspondence continued during the winter. The next spring she stopped in New York to see her sister at the hospital and spent a week in the city. On April 15, 1912, I called on her in her apartment hotel. We took a walk on that lovely evening in the park, between the Hudson and Riverside Drive. It was there and then that I realized how much we loved each other. I proposed to her and we pledged our troth.

The next morning I called on her early, and as we walked down Riverside Drive we saw a paper that announced the tragic loss of the Titanic, after striking an iceberg in the North Atlantic. But even this dreadful news did not dampen our joy. It was a beautiful spring day, the leaves were beginning to show in the trees and all seemed well with the world. We sent telegrams to our mothers, telling them of our happiness. That night we attended a performance of Tristan and Isolde.

Before Mary left for Boston we told the Auchinclosses and Ned Park our good news, and no one could have greeted it more cordially. We had a fine dinner at the Auchinclosses, with our health celebrated in French champagne.

We made plans to go to Duluth that summer, and we agreed that our engagement would necessarily be a long one. I did no work for the rest of the time that Mary stayed in the city, and we had a blissful few days until she took the train for Woods Hole. We went to Tiffany's and I bought Mary her engagement ring, but did not tell her that as a result I only had thirty dollars in my bank account! Shortly after Mary left, a beautiful leather-bound, Chapman's Edition set of Dickens arrived from Boston; Mary's engagement present to me. This was always our prize library possession, and increased my preference for Dickens as a storyteller. Alas! The leather bindings were not the same after more than forty years on our bookshelves.

In July we met and took a train for Duluth. It was a dear welcome we got from mother and the girls when we reached the home on East Third Street. They found that the glowing accounts of Mary's beautiful features and figure, her lovely golden hair, her little hands and feet, that I had tried to describe in my letters, had not done her justice, and they all fell in love with her. Picnics on the lakeshore and on the Point, with the culinary masterpieces of planked white fish by Lou Barton and Lucius, who came up from the mine in Wisconsin, were some of the good things that the family did for us. Eunice was especially concerned that Mary should be aware of my idiosyncrasies, and cautioned her against sneezing, after Mary had performed her usual twenty times!

By this time we were both convinced that a long engagement was the last thing we wanted, and come what may, we planned for a September wedding. I had the promise of a lucrative obstetrical case the latter part of September, and Dr. Adrian Lambert was turning a lot of work my way. The future looked promising to us as we looked at it through rosy colored glasses. September 26th was the date we chose for the wedding. Miss Sarah Fay, for whom Mary had worked several years as secretary and manager in her home, had invited us to hold the wedding reception in her old colonial house in the famous rose garden, after the wedding ceremony in the Church of the Messiah where Mary's father had been the rector before he died, as a young man of thirty-six. Mother Neales and mother Whipple promised to be there; James, Mary's brother, was to give her away; Margaret Neales was maid of honor. Lucius was to have been best man, but a shotgun accident prevented his coming. So I asked Johnnie St. John to take his place, for he was as close a friend as I had at that time.

On the 25th mother came to New York, and with her and the wedding party, we took the Fall River boat for Woods Hole. We reached Woods Hole on a typically perfect Cape morning - cool, clear, without a cloud in the sky.

The service was a very dear one in the church with so many associations, and was conducted by Father Cheeney, a former associate and close friend of Father Neales. The wedding breakfast at Miss Fay's home, with uncounted roses from the surrounding rose garden, was delightfully done.

With plenty of rice and roses thrown at us, Mary and I left for Middleborough where we got the Boston train for New York. We had decided secretly that in doing over the little fourth floor apartment, we would prepare it for our homecoming. To this home we came at 66 East 77th Street. Mary had chosen the golden grass wallpaper for the living room, and we had sent the various pieces of furniture that she had bought in Boston and that I had bought in New York to the apartment, so that we were set up for housekeeping as soon as we returned from our wedding trip in Manchester, Vermont. There we took a room in a house near the Dumont Clarks. I had promised to act as obstetrician for Mrs. Clark, who was expecting the arrival of their first child during the following week.

My experience in that capacity, although not serious, was rather trying because of the prudish attitude of the patient and her husband. When I mentioned the necessity of an obstetrical examination, it resulted in a flight to the attic on the lady's part, and a resort to prayer on the husband's part. When I told Mary of my difficulties, she thought it was a great joke and laughed merrily, to the extent that she made me see the humor of it and helped me survive the delivery, which came off without complications. But this experience and two later ones, that were no fault of mine, convinced me that obstetrics was not my branch of medicine, and ended my career in that field.

In April of 1913, Dr. Blake asked me to special a patient of his who lived in Islip, Long Island. He was a Harvard undergraduate who had been operated on for a severe streptococcus infection of his throat and neck, and had developed a septicemia, with positive blood cultures. After a long consultation at the Presbyterian where Dr. Blake had operated on him, it was decided that the best chance the boy had was to take him to his Islip home, where his father had a large estate and a house with outdoor sleeping porches. This was long before the days of the antibiotics when a blood stream streptococcus infection was usually fatal.

For more than two months I would take a five o'clock train for Islip, after rushing from the Englewood Hospital where I was the pathologist. This would get me to the Knapp's about seven, for a very good dinner following my examination of the patient, for Mr. Knapp was an epicure and they had plenty of fresh vegetables and fruit on their estate. For several weeks I would find Theodore having had a chill that afternoon, followed by a high fever, but with a ravenous appetite, oddly enough. This was fully satisfied with steak or roast beef, vegetables and fruit topped off with a pint of the best French champagne.

It was this food and fresh air that kept the patient going, and kept the courage and assurance of his father undaunted. Mr. Knapp was one of the most intelligent, charming men that I have ever known. His nightly review and discussion of his son's progress was as good as any clinician's. The boy did get well, notwithstanding the fact that he developed a suppurative knee joint which I aspirated eighteen times. He later joined the Navy in World War II, and at that time had perfect use of his knee; the examiners did not see the scars of the puncture marks I had made.

It was this spring that we expected the first addition to our family, and as June approached I became anxious to finish my job in Islip and planned to make my last visit during the first week in June. On Sunday, June 1st, Mary and Margaret and I went for a drive before I was to leave for Islip. There was no indication that day that anything was starting, but the next morning, about two o'clock, I had a telephone call from Johnnie St. John, who was living around the corner from us, telling me that Mary had called him and he had found that labor had started. He had called George Ryder, my old friend and Mary's obstetrician. I told John that I would take the first milk train to New York to reach New York by eight o'clock. When I arrived in the apartment and walked into the bedroom, there was my Mary with a happy smile on her face holding a wee daughter. Was I surprised! Neither John nor George had expected such rapid action. There never was a lovelier mother or a lovelier little daughter.

Footnotes

1. **C. Irving Fisher (1847-1924)**

   A graduate of Harvard Medical School, he began his career as the Port Physician of Boston. He later became the superintendent of the Massachusetts State Hospital. After eight years he resigned to assume the position of the Head of the Presbyterian Hospital until 1914.

2. **Anna C. Maxwell (1852-1929)**

   As Dean of American nurses she has been called "the American Florence Nightingale". Maxwell was the inspiring spirit of the School of Nursing in the Presbyterian Hospital. During the war with Spain (1898) Maxwell, together with 160 assistants invaded Camp Thomas in Georgia where they successfully reduced the typhoid death rate to a record number. She was told: "When you came we did not know what to do with you. Now we do not know what to do without you."

3. **Theodore C Janeway (1872-1917)**

   The son of Edward Janeway, the Dean of New York University and Bellevue Hospital Medical College and a graduate of the P & S of Columbia University. He wrote a book about blood pressure and designed the first satisfactory apparatus for blood pressure measurement at the bedside. In 1914 he was invited to the Johns Hopkins Medical School to take the previous chair held by Dr. William Osler.

4. **William G. MacCallum (-)**

   Professor of Pathology at the P & S of Columbia University, best known for his *Textbook of Pathology*.

5. **John English McWhorter (1875-1936)**

   A graduate of P & S of Columbia University in 1898. Devoting his entire time for pathology of surgical diseases, he contributed the first photographic observations ever made of earliest angiogenesis and first heartbeats in the chick embryo.

6. **Edwards Park (1878-1969)**

   A graduate of P & S of Columbia University in 1905. While a Professor of Pediatrics at Yale University, his studies on rickets proved the healing power of cod liver oil and sunlight.

Chapter Nine

Junior Attending
1915 - 1921

The next spring I was appointed to the surgical staff of the Presbyterian, as a junior attending, and began active operative work again. This meant that I had a good deal of the emergency work to do, with a great deal of assisting the house surgeons. But I still worked in the surgical pathology laboratory with Bill Clarke, and continued as instructor to the surgical clerks.

The summer of 1915 we rented a very simple cottage on Corn Hill at the east end of the Cape. Mother Whipple and Eunice joined us, and we had a lot of mother's good cooking, some of it of the Persian variety. Maynam [1], our daughter, was a very active two-year old child; she kept us busy trying to prevent her rolling down the steep hill into the bay below. One of my happy memories is connected with her excitement at watching and hearing the "tooty train" as she sat on my shoulder at the top of the hill, watching the daily train coming around the bend. We have some charming pictures of her, au naturelle, on the Bay Shore looking at the shell of a horseshoe crab that she had found on the beach.

On December 13, 1915, Allen Jr. arrived; a long, big baby. We were not as agreed as to his name, as in the case of his sister, for I thought it was not fair to give him the name of Oldfather when he had nothing to say about it. But after two weeks, his mother persuaded me to the idea, and so that name he has borne ever since. But his first name has had variations. Mum, as we now began calling Mary, used her pet name of

Sonny Bun for Allen; this changed to Son Bun; Mary called him Bumps, and he has been called that by the family ever since. Because of his long legs and jolly smile, he was sometimes called "The Boob", but I resented this and predicted that he would turn into a handsome boy, and sure enough, before he was four years old mum had a pastel portrait made of him which we have always cherished.

World War I had started in 1914 and was the chief topic in the papers and with everyone we knew. At first the well-organized German army gained great victories over the French, the British and the Russians. But the invasion of Belgium was their first mistake, for it started the great prejudice against the Germans in this country, increasing as time went on. The splendid resistance that the French and the British put up, though with terrible losses, was tremendously admired. For two years there was a strong feeling that this was a European calamity, and that we should maintain a neutral position, although Wilson's attitude of watchful waiting was increasingly resented. The submarine warfare of the Germans, with the sinking of ships on the free seas, created a mounting anger in this country. When the Lusitania was sunk with many Americans lost, loud and angry protests were heard from all parts of the country. I can remember the afternoon that the specials appeared announcing that tragedy, and meeting Evan Evans, who said that this was the end of neutrality. The Lusitania disaster was the final cause of this country's declaring war on Germany in April of 1917. Of course many of the officials in the government and men in the know realized that our joining the Allies was inevitable, so that a certain amount of preparedness had been going on. But once war was declared it was amazing how quickly things began to move.

One of the things that was most important was the organization of hospitals to go overseas with the expeditionary forces. A number of prominent surgeons had gone to France and England during the previous year to help in the care of the Allied troops. But as soon as war was declared, several of the university hospitals began organizing and equipping their units for overseas work, and the Presbyterian was one of the first to do so. At the first meeting for this purpose which was held at the College of P & S all the younger men on the staff of the Presbyterian enlisted, I among them. Within a few days the official appointments to the Medical Corps of the United States Army arrived. Like the younger surgeons, I was appointed a First Lieutenant. But within ten days this was re-called at the insistence of Dean Lambert, who declared that I was essential to the teaching in the medical school. This caused me no end of resentment at first, but an explanation of it by several members of the faculty and at the hospital, together with the fact that we were expecting the arrival of another child in June and my realization of how hard it would be for Mary, reconciled me to the edict of the dean, especially when he said that there would be plenty of opportunities to go overseas later. But that never came, although I applied and was told that I would be appointed a few weeks before the war ended.

That June the 23rd, dear Bill arrived, a beautiful baby with a shock of dark hair and deep blue eyes. But before he came we had a siege of measles in the house on Madison Avenue and 86th Street. Maynam was desperately sick with a complicating pneumonia. Howard Mason was away at the time, but we had a skillful and constantly encouraging pediatrician in Fred Bartlett. At the time when things looked hopeless, Howard returned to the city and helped pull Maynam through the crisis. It was only two days after this that Mary had to go to the Sloane Hospital for Bill's arrival.

We had a Scotch maid at that time that worshipped the ground that Bumps walked on. She taught him to sing Scotch ditties and to dance with her in Highland flings. While the worst of the measles was going on, he, having recovered quickly, spent part of his unobserved time in throwing some of the family flat silver out of the third story window into the back yard. Not all of it was recovered.

That summer we went to Wilton, Connecticut, for the first time. We had been urged to do so by Sally Middlebrook, the aunt of Marriana Richards, one of our and Arch Strong's close friends. She was the first citizen of Wilton, and with her brother lived in one of the loveliest houses in the town. As we were driving to their home, we saw the goods and chattels of a house by the side of the road. These belonged to a strange character that had refused to pay her taxes on a house with several small dollhouses around it. She later pitched her tent on the east side of an old cemetery, still refusing to pay her taxes.

We rented a charming old cottage with a fine fireplace in the living room and an old-fashioned flower garden. This was our introduction to Wilton that became a part of our lives for many years. Wilton then was a typical old-fashioned Connecticut town. It had no trolley, but the country store was the gathering place for interesting old characters. Among them were John and Sally Scofield. He was the town butcher and peddled his meat from his wagon. This wagon Mary was called upon to drive with Sally when "John aint a peddlin' today." This meant that he was recovering from one of his periodic benders. On one such episode he appeared in front of our cottage in his stocking feet and wearing a small barrel on his head.

Our summer home then was a newly acquired old farmhouse on Grumman Hill known as the Weed Farm. After our second year in Wilton we had found the house with 28 acres, more or less, of land. When we had the land surveyed later, we found we had 38 acres! The house, which was built by the Weed family in 1830, was unfurnished, so that we had to scout around during the next year in getting necessary furniture and equipment. We had bought the first station wagon - a model T Ford - that was seen in Wilton. We have a precious picture of Bill, then only fifteen months old, trying to crank the car. When I first bought the station wagon and was driving in the barn, not knowing the technique of the pedal mechanism, I pushed the wrong pedal and drove the car through the back of the barn.

Footnotes

1.   **Maynam**

Maynam was another name for Dr. Whipple's daughter, Mary. She also had the nickname of 'Sis'.

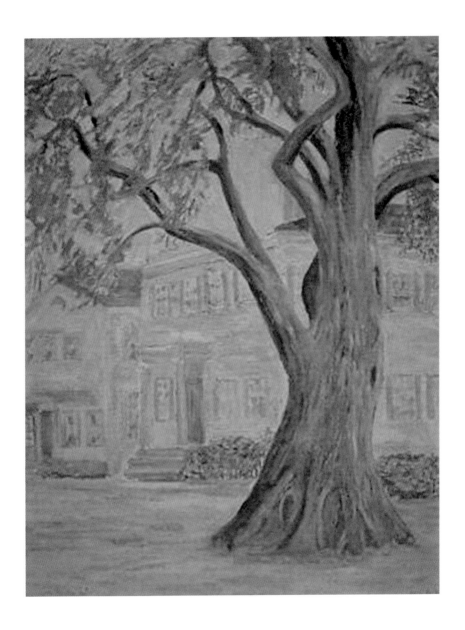

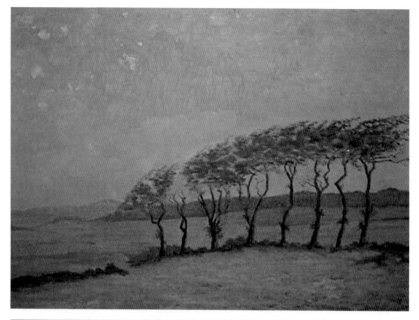

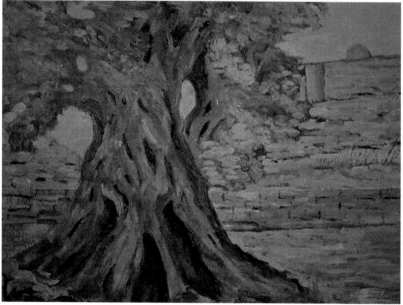

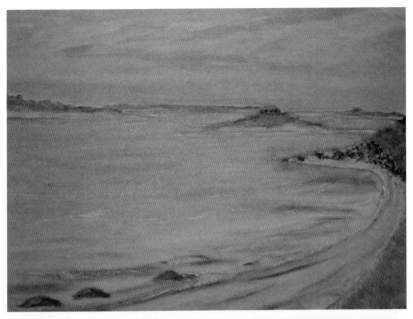

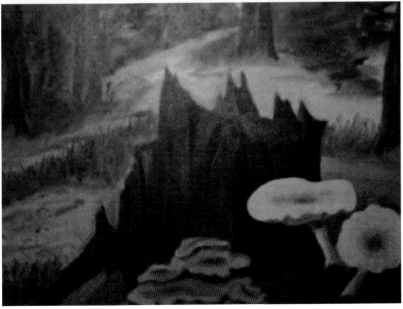

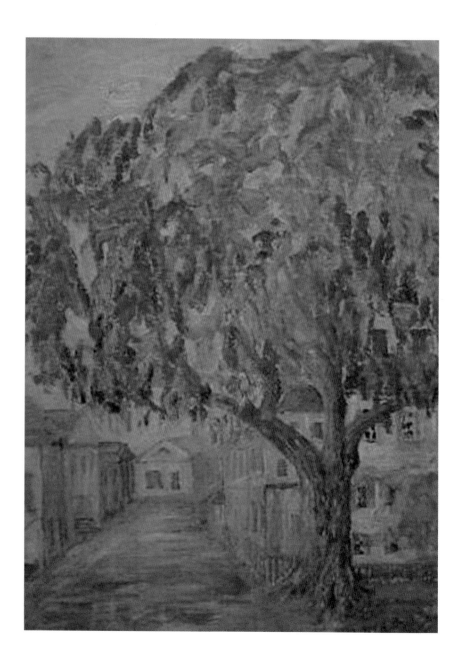

Chapter Ten

Director of Surgery

1921 - 1930

The year we bought the Wilton house we moved to Beekham Place, at the end of 50th Street and the East River. There we lived for two years, except for the summer in New York. It was in the basement kitchen of this house that a very important meeting was held on a winter evening. The men attending it were Hans Zinsser, Bill Clarke, John and myself. A crisis had been reached in the medical school, following the resignation of Dean Lambert. The man who had been gunning for the job was an astute politician, but opposed to any reform in the conduct of the school or the Presbyterian. Many of us were very opposed to this man getting the deanship. At this meeting in our kitchen, Zinsser proposed Bill Darrach as the man who could command the respect of the faculty and the help of Ed Harkness, his Yale classmate. We all agreed to this, and at the next meeting of the faculty, Darrach was proposed and was elected over the man who thought that he had the appointment in the bag.

Because of Darrach's friendship with Harkness, he was able to make some radical changes in the policies of the school and hospital. It was decided that full time appointments for the heads of the medical and surgical departments should be made. In the spring of 1921 I was offered such a full time appointment at Columbia and at Yale. The decision as to which of these offers I should accept was a most difficult one. Mary and I, together with Warfield Longcope [1] and his wife (he had been offered the professorship in medicine at both places), went to New

Haven to look the place over. We were given a very cordial reception, with a luncheon, with every attention shown us.

But when we returned I was still in a quandary until Bill Darrach and Hans Zinsser convinced me that I should stay with Columbia. So I was appointed Professor of Surgery at Columbia and Director of the Surgical Service at the Presbyterian, and began my duties on July 1st, 1921 and held them for 25 years until I retired in 1946 at the required age of 65.

One of the first and most trying duties was to reorganize the surgical staff at the Presbyterian. I had nice letters of resignation from the older men of the staff who did not want to embarrass me by not resigning and who did not care to go on a full time basis. It was especially hard to have Adrian Lambert go, for he had been such a good friend of mine. But later I was able to persuade him to take charge of the surgical service on the first division at the Bellevue Hospital, a teaching division under Columbia. With a clean slate I appointed the younger men with whom I had worked and knew intimately: Johnnie St. John and Barclay Parsons [2] on the first surgical division, and Hugh Auchincloss and John Hanford [3] on the second division.

It was at this time that I started the residency program at the Presbyterian, the first in any of the hospitals in New York. The first four whom I appointed were Harold Harvey [4] and Larry Sloan [5], both of them former house surgeons, Richmond Moore [6], who had trained at the Brigham in Boston and at the Rockefeller Institute in New York, and Jerome Webster [7], who had worked with Halsted at the Hopkins and had been with the Pekin Union Memorial for three years. All four of these men turned out to be first class, leading surgeons in their special fields which they developed at the Presbyterian. They have all retired at the age of sixty-five, though still active now in private practice.

Soon after I started as Surgical Director, one of my senior interns Harry Murray, now one of the leading psychiatrists in Boston, came to see me after he had returned from a vacation in England. He said he knew that I was anxious to get a man to do the neurological surgery at the hospital, and told me that he thought that he had found the very man for the job, and that I ought to get in touch with him immediately as he was coming to the States shortly. He said the surgeon's name was Wilder Penfield [8], that he had been a Rhodes scholar after graduating from Princeton, that he had graduated from the Hopkins Medical School and had had a residency in neurological surgery at the Queens Square Hospital in London and had worked with the famous physiologist, Sherrington, in Oxford. This all sounded most promising, so I cabled Penfield asking him to see me when he came through New York. This he did and I was very much impressed with him, both with his personality and his qualifications for the job. I made him a good offer, but was not able to offer him a lucrative salary. He said he was very much interested, but that he could not give a definite answer until he had gone to Detroit, where he had been offered a somewhat similar job, but at a much higher salary. I asked him to come back to see me if he did not take the Detroit offer. He said he certainly would.

I knew that the superintendent of the Ford Hospital, who had made Penfield the offer, had been in charge of the Peace Ship that Henry Ford had sent to bring the boys out of the trenches by Christmas. This made me feel fairly sure that Penfield would come again. When he went to the Ford Hospital, he was given a big luncheon and much attention. Before he was to leave, the superintendent asked him to stop in his office, and there he asked Penfield what he was especially interested in. When Penfield said he wanted to continue his research in the field of neurology and neurological surgery, the man said, "That's fine, just tell us what you want investigated and we will do it for you." Penfield reached for his hat and said, "I appreciate very much the kind reception that you have given me, but I will not be able to accept the offer." He took the next train for New York and came to see me to ask if my offer to him was still good, because he would like very much to join our group. He became one of the most admired and beloved members of our staff, and worked with us for the next seven years.

I told him that the only thing that he lacked was some experience in general surgery, and I thought he should have it as a background for his neurological surgery. He said he realized this only too well and would appreciate the opportunity of getting it. So I appointed him to the second division to work with Hugh, and I personally gave him a lot of major surgery, assisting him or having him assisting me. He quickly demonstrated his ability and serious interest in the work. He soon established a laboratory for research in neurological surgery, and appointed a young lad from Iowa, Bill Cone, who soon made a name for himself. But in 1928, when Wilder was offered the directorship of the newly built and heavily endowed Neurological Institute in Montreal, I had to advise him to take the offer, which he did, taking Bill Cone with him, to the great loss of Columbia and the new Medical Center.

During the years at the old Presbyterian, before we moved uptown to the new Medical Center, we were a small, very congenial group, knowing one another intimately and able to understand each other. The picture, which I have and most highly prize, is of the surgical staff taken in 1924. Those in the picture, seated from left to right, were Penfield, Auchincloss, Bill Clarke, myself, St. John, Van Beuren and Parsons. Standing were Bill Cone, Beverley Smith, John Hanford, Virginia Frantz, Louis Bauman, Doris Ryker (head nurse in the operating room), Anne Penfield (head anesthetist), Carl Janssen, Rudy Schullinger, Frank Meleney, Dave Bull, and Purdy Scott.

We developed good ideas. One of these was organizing the follow-up clinic, the first, not only in New York, but also in the country. Another was the development of the Unit Record System with the medical service, again a first in the city. Still another was the holding of regular surgical conferences once a week to discuss the errors in diagnosis, the mistakes in technique and the infections of clean wounds and deaths, if any had occurred during the past week.

Our relations with the Medical Service were most cordial and constructive, largely because of the appointment of Bill Palmer [9] as Professor of Medicine and Director of the Medical Service at the Presbyterian. His staff included some of the best young men at the hospital before he came from the Hopkins with several of his top men

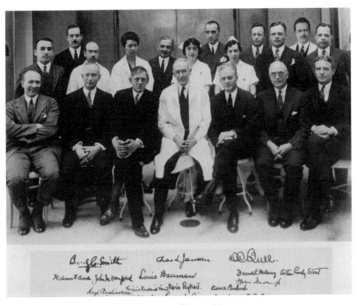

The Presbyterian surgical staff in 1924.

from that hospital. This fine spirit between the two services continued when we moved uptown for as long as I worked there.

Beginning in 1925, plans for the new medical center began to develop, and soon blueprints started to appear to be reviewed by the different departments. We had a very energetic man in charge of the building program, but his previous training in psychiatry, oddly enough, had not helped him to understand the needs of the various departments, nor how to get along with the men heading them. In fact, for two years he was a constant pain in the neck to those of us who had ideas of what was needed in the greatly expanded hospital, and it was a constant battle to make sure that our ideas, not his, would go from the blueprint stage into bricks and mortar. Strangely enough, when he was replaced and went to take charge of a mental hospital, he never held a grudge against me, but continued to send me Christmas books, which he had privately printed, and extracts from an astonishing variety of his favorite authors from Plato to Mark Twain.

After 1921 we lived in several places, and for two years in 319 East 68th Street. This was a four-story house, with lots of room, for we needed it then. We had three pianos, separate rooms for the boys and Eunice and Sis in another. At that time we had a Swiss girl, Bertha, working for us who turned out to be a jewel. Mary taught her how to cook, and she became a real culinary artist. On Saturdays Mary would load edibles, blankets, and Sandy, our wirehaired fox terrier, in the station wagon and go to Wilton for the weekend. I used to come up later, but frequently had to rush back to the hospital in response to an urgent telephone call.

I should have said earlier that the fall and winter after I had accepted the professorship, Mary and the children spent this time in Wilton. We had a Scotch couple and their small boy living in the house. The man was the gardener and handy man. We had two cows that supplied us with all the milk we could use. Mary always said the most exciting job she had that winter was skimming the milk pans for Jersey cream in the morning as soon as she came downstairs. That winter was a cold one and the Model T station wagon was difficult to start. On more than one occasion I had to pour ether into the carburetor and hike up the rear end of the car before I could get the engine started. When I was not there Mary would have to call the Gregory boys, the Ford mechanics in town, to get the car started. Sometimes even they could not get the old thing going, and the kids would have to miss school in the village.

In the summer of 1925 Mary and I went to Europe with the Society of Clinical Surgery. We sailed on the Italian liner the Duillo, a very comfortable ship with a splendid cuisine. The company we were with was delightful; most of the men were the heads of surgical departments in university clinics and medical schools whom I had known well at the various surgical meetings. Quite a number of the wives were in the party, and we came to know them well, as one does on such a trip. The Gibbons of Philadelphia were our closest friends. I played chess with John on the ship and on the trains, and did not mind being defeated by him for he played with skill and debonairly.

We landed in Naples and spent three days sightseeing in places like Pompeii and the fine museums. From there we went to Rome and stayed at the Hotel Russie, a delightful hotel on the Pizza del Populo, opposite a church that had charming little statues on the edges of its roof. The few days we spent in Rome were too few to see so many of the places we wanted to visit. The men attended two of the leading clinics, where we saw some good and some bad surgery. That was my first acquaintance with Bastienelli [10], a very charming and aristocratic Italian surgeon. My subsequent contacts with him were much more interesting and will be told later in this story.

From Rome we motored to Florence, then to Bologna where we visited a most interesting orthopedic clinic that was housed in an old monastery and directed by a striking character, Professor Putti [11], a very clever orthopedic surgeon and a talented sculptor. To see him remodel a knee joint that had been immobile for months was a sight to admire. The library and record room of the clinic had been the refectory of the old monastery. It contained paintings by some of the most famous artists of the 14th and 15th centuries. In Bologna we also visited the oldest anatomical amphitheater and saw the cloisters of the ancient medical school of the university with the names of famous physicians, like William Harvey, the discoverer of the circulation, on their university shields painted on the ceiling.

From there we went to Venice and were entertained by a very picturesque figure, Professor Giordano [12], a former pupil of Billroth. He had been the mayor of Venice and was at that time a Senator, so that he was well known everywhere. His every gesture was obeyed. He conducted us to all the best-known places, took us in his powerboat to see the famous glass works and lace factories in the Lido, and there gave us an elaborate luncheon at the Excelsior-Palace Hotel. The surgeons attended his operative clinic, which was unique in many ways, for he used the same technique that Billroth had used in Vienna some fifty years before. He had a magnificent white beard that came well down to his chest. In the operating room he wore no mask, but his beard was hidden in what would well have served as a feedbag. He was quick in his gestures, and when he turned his head suddenly to answer our questions, out would pop some part of his imprisoned whiskers, requiring the disturbing attentions of one of the nurses in replacing the errant beaver in the feedbag.

We saw him remove a very large spleen from a young man whose history and laboratory findings made the diagnosis of chronic lymphatic leukemia very obvious - a condition in no way benefited by the removal of the spleen. We asked Giordano why he was removing the spleen. He said, "It bothers the patient, he wants it out."

From Venice we went to the Dolomites and spent four days in the grand mountains and valleys of that amazing country. I lost my favorite Dunhill pipe in motoring up one of the steep roads, but was able to find it when I walked back to one of the other cars that was following us. More about this later. We then traveled into the Austrian Alps and stopped in Innsbruck, and from there to Zurich to attend the clinics of the well known surgeons in those cities. Then to Berne and Lucerne where we saw Professor Roux [13] do some remarkable chest surgery. One of his patients was a young woman of twenty who was having part of the ribs of her chest removed. This was done under local anesthesia; frequently Roux would ask her if she felt pain or were getting tired, and would then tell the nurse to give her more champagne.

From Berne we went to Strasbourg and were entertained by the famous surgeon Leriche [14], much the best surgeon we had seen in our travels. He was bold, with an active imagination, and had very fine aseptic technique, much of which he had learned, he said, from Halsted in Baltimore whom he admired greatly. The Leriches gave the Society a very fine luncheon in their home. Champagne was served from pitcher and was delicious. Mary's French, and John Gibbon's, got fluent, and he said to her, "Mary, if you take more of this delicious stuff, you will be talking Spanish and I won't be able to talk at all."

To Paris, where we had a delightful week, I was more interested in the city's many attractions than I was in French surgery, for what I saw of it was fast, careless, and with bad technique, and too many organs were removed with improper diagnoses. Mary and I did a lot of sightseeing together, visiting places that we had known before. The party went to Brussels, but Mary and I left Paris for Le Havre, where we took the Duilio back to New York. It did not take us more than a couple of hours after arriving there to get to Wilton and the dear ones. How glad we were to come home!

Two of my closest friends, Arch Strong and Jim Corscaden, had taken lessons on the cello. In 1924 they persuaded me to join them in their lessons with their teacher, Bedrich Vaska, whom we called the Maestro. All three of us were busy doctors, with little time to practice the cello, but the Maestro was understanding and patient, and tolerated our amateurish attempts. But we had great fun with him and with the poor music we produced. When Mary and I were returning on the Duilio, the cellist in the trio that played at dinner and in the evenings, had an Italian instrument made in Genoa in the latter part of the seventeenth century. It was a beautiful cello with a lovely tone. I asked the cellist if he would care to sell it. He said no, but that if he did change his mind, he would let me know. Some five months later he came to see me with his cello. We had it appraised and I bought it; it became one of my prized possessions, even if it were not appreciated so much by the rest of the family who suffered under my playing it. I only wish that I could have practiced both surgery and the cello.

In 1928 the new Medical Center, the combined College of Physicians and Surgeons and the Presbyterian Hospital, the Sloane Hospital, the Babies and the Neurological, the Vanderbuilt Clinic, and later the Eye Institute and Maxwell Hall for the Nurses, was opened. Miss Anna Maxwell was the first patient to enter the Harkness Pavilion where she died a few weeks later, beloved and revered by all the nurses and doctors. The Nurses Hall was named for her.

We had to look for a place to live near the new center. At first we thought of buying a house on Haven Avenue, but we were worried that the neighborhood was rapidly changing and that it would be a considerable risk. So we rented an apartment on Haven Avenue, overlooking the Hudson River. The magnificent view compensated for some of the deficiencies of the apartment. Here we lived until we bought the house on Fieldston Road in Riverdale.

Before the hospital moved uptown, there had been considerable doubt as to whether we would be able to fill it as it was four times the old bed capacity, with all the affiliated hospitals. But within three months, all the beds in the several units were filled and a waiting list was started.

The Presbyterian Hospital had one great advantage in that the staff that had been reorganized in 1921 did not have to be changed, but moved to the new building without any difficulty. The best traditions of the old hospital were brought to the new one. This was a great blessing, for the New York Hospital had quite the opposite experience when it was moved from 15th Street to the new site on East 68th Street. A new surgical staff was appointed under an imported surgical director, with no regard for the fine old traditions and portraits of the second oldest hospital in America. There was a very serious break in the relations between the new and the old; especially the former graduates of the hospital and the feud lasted for twenty years or more.

Of course there was plenty of readjusting to do in the work of the hospitals and the medical school, but the advantage of having them in such close proximity became immediately apparent. All the trekking between East 70th Street and West 59th Street was eliminated. The groups from the school and the hospitals met every day in the common dining room and were soon talking the same language and understanding better the problems in common.

The residency-training program in surgery was developing most satisfactorily, and we were getting a fine group of men applying for the positions, not only from the College of P & S, but also from other medical schools, especially Harvard. The animal hospital and the experimental operating facilities in the College offered new opportunities for work in experimental surgery and more of the attendings and residents were making use of it. Frank Meleney [15] had developed the first laboratory in bacteriology in any surgical service in this country and was especially interested in the study of surgical infections. Louis Bauman [16] had continued his work in chemical studies of surgical patients and Jerome Webster had started a training program in plastic surgery that soon became known as the leading center for residency training in that specialty. Hugh Auchincloss continued his splendid work in the surgery of the hand and breast tumors. Johnnie St. John and Harold Harvey had begun their work in the study of the lesions of the stomach and duodenum. Carl Janssen [17], who had come to us from Belgium at the end of the war, a brilliant and cultured surgeon, was making a reputation for his surgery of the colon and rectum. Barclay Parsons and Larry Sloan, with Bill Palmer in medicine, had developed a unique thyroid clinic and we were getting more thyroid patients than any other group.

We continued our studies in gall bladder and biliary tract disease, and I started the Spleen Clinic with Pete Rousselot [18] and Pat Elliot [19], two of our able recently graduated residents. We had Bill Thompson and Frank Hanger with us in this project from the medical service. These all developed into what were called combined clinics, in which men from the medical, surgical and pathological services worked together as a team which studied patients before treatment, decided on the best treatment and, after they had left the hospital, saw them as a group in the follow-up clinic. This was one of the most constructive developments that had ever been made in the hospital and medical school. It meant that the medical students did not think of diseases of the thyroid and spleen and such lesions as ulcers as medical or surgical, but rather as entities, some of which needed one form of therapy; others, another. It also broke down the barriers between the various services that had not previously seen results of other forms of treatment.

Footnotes

1. **Warfield T. Longcope (-1953)**
    A graduate of Johns Hopkins in 1901 and for many years a medical director and Bard Professor of the Practice of Medicine. Later on he became a Professor of Medicine and Physician-in-Chief at the Johns Hopkins Hospital.

2. **William Parsons (1889-1973)**
    A graduate of P & S of Columbia in 1914. Shortly before America entered WW II, Parsons joined with 35 doctors opposed to a plan to supply food to the conquered Europe; they wrote to President Franklin D. Roosevelt that the plan, however

humane, "would prolong, rather than cure, the suffering of the conquered peoples of Europe". He became President of the New York Academy of Medicine (1951-1953), and Chairman of the Board of Directors of the American Field Service Committee.

3. **John Hanford (-1973)**

    A graduate of New York University in 1909 who occupied several positions at the Presbyterian Hospital and Columbia University. His special interest was the management of tuberculous cervical lymphadenopathy.

4. **Harold Harvey (1893-1973)**

    A graduate of P & S of Columbia University in 1925 and a member of its surgical faculty until retirement. His areas of interest included peritonitis, surgical infections, peptic ulcer disease and cancer of the stomach.

5. **Lawrence Wells Sloan (1896-)**

    A graduate of Harvard Medical School in 1925. He completed his surgical residency at the P & S Hospitals and continued there as a faculty. His areas of interest included thyroid diseases and spinal analgesia.

6. **Richmond L. Moore (1896-)**

    A graduate of Harvard University in 1922. After a residency at the Rockefeller Institute for medical research he joined the surgical faculty at the Presbyterian Hospital. From 1954 he was an attending in thoracic surgery at the V.A. Hospital, Bronx, New York.

7. **Jerome Pierce Webster (1888-1974)**

    A graduate of Johns Hopkins School of Medicine in 1914. Shortly before the United States entered WWI he was sent to Berlin to inspect camps of prisoner-of-war. Three years later, after a residency at the Johns Hopkins he went to China as the first surgical resident of the new Peking Union Medical College. During WWII he organized plastic surgery centers for the US Army. In 1954 he became a consultant surgeon and professor emeritus at the P & S of Columbia. An avid collector of books, he donated his library of more than 5,000 books, known as the Jerome P. Webster Library of Plastic Surgery, to the Columbia-Presbyterian Medical Center.

8. **Wilder Penfield (1891-1976)**

    A graduate of Johns Hopkins in 1918. He moved to McGill University, Montreal in 1928 where he pioneered a center for brain surgery. He attempted mapping of the brain and surgical treatment of epilepsy.

9. **Walter Walker Palmer (1888-1950)**

A graduate of the Harvard University in 1910 and a Professor of Medicine at the P & S of Columbia. He carried out pioneer studies in acid-base balance, the thyroid glands, diabetes and nephritis. He was credited with the development of one of the first accurate methods for determination of hemoglobin.

10. **Ricardo Di Raffaelle Bastienelli (1863-1961)**

A renowned Italian surgeon. He was the general director of "dell'Istituto Regina Elena" for the study and cure of tumors in Rome, and the founder of "di Clinica Chirurgica". He was acknowledged by surgeons like Lord Moynihan, Harvey Cushing, and the brothers Mayo. He became a pilot at the age of 68, at which time he had an accident with a tree that led to minor scalp laceration.

11. **Vittorio Putti (1880-1940)**

A master of orthopedic surgery and a bibliophile. From the age of 30 the chief surgeon of Istituto Orthopedico Rizzole and a Professor of Orthopedics at the University of Bologna. Putti assembled a remarkable private collection of medical books and instruments, which was later donated to the Istituto Orthopedico Rizzoli in Bologna.

12. **David Giordano (1864-1954)**

An Italian surgeon best known for proposing the transglabellar surgical approach to the pituitary gland. He was a founding member of the International Society of Surgery (1924).

13. **Cesar Roux (1857-1934)**

A Professor of Surgery in Lausanne, Switzerland. Inspired by his mentor Theodor Kocher of Berne, Theodor Billroth and Richard von Volkmann, he is best known for the Roux-en-Y loop (1892), the first esophagojejunostomy (1904) and the first adrenalectomy (1926).

14. **Rene Henri Marie Leriche (1879-1955)**

A French vascular surgeon who was Professor of Surgery in Strasbourg and Lyon before becoming a Professor of the College de France in Paris in 1936. He is best known for his description of the syndrome caused by incomplete obstruction of the bifurcation of the aorta, which is named after him. He was an early advocate of sympathectomy but anticipated already in the 1920s that the ideal treatment for arterial occlusion would be a vascular graft. Leriche's interest in pain was summarized in a monograph: *La Chirurgerie de la Douleur.*

15. Frank Lamont Meleney (1889-1963)

A graduate of P & S of Columbia in 1916. His chief contributions were in the field of clinical bacteriology and surgical infections. He wrote two books on surgical infections and the "synergistic soft tissue infection" is named after him.

16. Louis Bauman (-1954)

Received his M.D. in 1901. He joined P & S as a faculty where he was an assistant Professor of Clinical Surgery between 1930 and 1945.

17. Charles Janssen (1886-1941)

A Belgian surgeon who attended King Leopold. Janssen came to New York in 1923 and was affiliated with Columbia University and the Presbyterian Hospital. His earlier papers in Europe dealt with war wounds. In New York he excelled in colorectal surgery, obtaining excellent results with abdomino-perineal resection for the cancer of the rectum.

18. Louis M. Rousselot (1902-1974)

After surgical training at the Presbyterian Hospital he collaborated with Whipple at the Spleen Clinic where the syndrome of portal hypertension was better defined: patients with splenomegaly, esophageal varices, and ascites were discovered to have portal hypertension. Two papers by Rousselot and colleagues (1936, 1937) reported direct measurements of portal pressure paving the road towards future application of portacaval anastomoses into clinical practice. Rousselot was a founder member of the Society of University Surgeons, the Allen O. Whipple Surgical Society, the Society for Surgery of the Alimentary Tract, and the New York Society for Cardiovascular Surgery.

19. Robert Elliott (1906-1977)

A graduate of the P & S of Columbia University in 1932 and a Professor of Surgery in 1965. He became Associate Dean for the P & S and Assistant Vice-president for the Presbyterian Hospital between 1966-1972.

Chapter Eleven

Sabbatical in Europe

1930

By 1930 I had completed nine years of full time work as the Head of the Surgical Department and was entitled to a sabbatical leave. So we planned to go to Europe as a family. The last week after Christmas of '29 we sailed on the old Minnekahda, not a fashionable liner, but a comfortable one that met all our requirements. It was only a day or two before the boys had come to know the First Mate and had been in the Captain's quarters in the fo'castle watching the steering and charting. The first day out, mum and I were the only ones who did not feel the motion of the ship, but in a day or two the kids had found their sea legs and were having a fine time. The ship was not a fast one, but the ten days we were on it passed quickly.

We had purchased a new Ford, a handsome brown car with a special rear platform to hold the various bags and suitcases that we had to take with us in motoring through the countries we planned to visit. The boys got a great kick out of seeing the car hoisted aboard in a net and lowered to the hold below. Fortunately Bumps kept an accurate diary of the entire trip, and I shall have frequent quotations from it. Where quotation marks are used in this story, they mean excerpts from his diary.

"Boulogne, January 21st, 1930. We could not get the car from the boat, so we stayed at the Hotel Bristol and saw the fish market and the town."

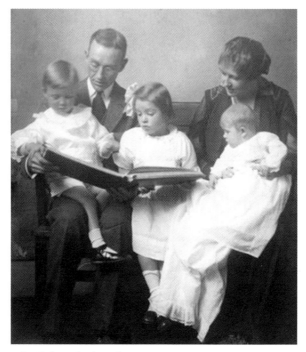

The Whipple family.

"January 22nd. Arrived at Amiens. Went to the cathedral and then to the Grand Hotel. The next morning saw the battlefields and the town of Montdidie. Left for Paris, 168 miles away, and arrived there that evening." As a matter of fact, we were not as calm as the diary would indicate, for it was after seven at night and we did not know where we were to stay. But we crossed to the Left Bank and found a pension, the Malherbe, on Rue de Vaugirard, where we stayed for a few days until we went to the Merciers where we had been recommended by the Stouts in New York. The Merciers were a typical Parisian family, living beyond Porte Maillot in Neuilly. Charles Mercier was a nephew of Cardinal Mercier, and had been a major in the Belgian Army during World War I. He had married a charming Parisienne who spoke perfect French. We made arrangements to have our meals with their family five days a week, when only French was to be spoken. Saturdays and Sundays we toured the surrounding cathedral towns within a radius of 200 kilometers, spending Saturday night in one of the towns.

These excursions proved to be most delightful and instructive, for we saw many of the cathedral towns with their wonderful churches, and saw the native French people, often very different and not so money-wise as the Parisians. At first the boys were reluctant to go to the cathedrals, for these were Catholic and on Sundays when we went to them, services were in progress. The kids thought it was very bad manners to go there while the people were at worship and did not realize that people went in and out of the church at all times, regardless of the service. The cathedrals that we thought were the most magnificent and interesting were in Amiens, Rheims and Rouen, but above all, Chartres. We went there five times and saw the wonderful glass in the cathedral in all seasons and in different lights.

I had decided that I did not want to see much of French surgery, which I had learned was very inferior to our own on the previous visit to Paris. So I thought it would be better to work in L'Ecole de Medicine, in Brumpt's laboratory, in the study of mycology, or moulds, in which I had done some work at the Presbyterian. They were very cooperative, giving me a desk with bacteriological equipment. I had brought with me some interesting strains of moulds, which we had recovered, we thought, from a patient on whom I had operated for a cyst of the liver. I continued to study this fungus in Brumpt's laboratory, under the guidance of M. Langeron. He was very agreeable, but he had a pronounced stutter, so that at first I had some difficulty in understanding his peculiar brand of French. But we became good friends and, although I did not make any startling discoveries, I did find that this particular fungus behaved in an entirely different way on French bread than on the New York bread on which I had previously grown it. M. Langeron easily explained it. He said the proportions of the ingredients in the two kinds of bread were different, and that the wheat in the standard Paris bread was different from that in New York.

Quite differently from the laboratories in America and England, when noon arrived everyone in the Paris Laboratory disappeared, no two workers going out together. I found a most attractive little restaurant to take the French dejeuner, a place called Michauds, on Rue Jacob not far from the laboratory. There I soon discovered a typical Parisian gourmet, who used to appear regularly with his demi-mondaine girlfriend; they would sit at the bar for an aperitif, which was always served them by the madame who sat at the casse. After the aperitif the girl would walk out of the side door, and the gourmet would always take a table near where I sat. I soon noticed that he was well aware of the best dishes and wines of the place, so that I often ordered the same things.

Several years later when I was in Paris, I went to Michauds for a mid-day meal and took my old seat, expecting to see the old gourmet, but he did not appear. The Madame was still there at her place behind the casse. I went up to her after paying l'addition, and asked her where the distinguished gourmet was. She threw up her hands and said, "Oh mon Dieu monsieur! Quelle domage, il etait mon mari, il est mort!" Some two years later on my return from a trip to Shiraz, I had to stop in Paris to see Mr. Nemazee, and went to Rue Jacob, expecting to have another dejeuner at Michauds, but I could not find it. On asking one of the men across the way what had become of the restaurant he shrugged his shoulders and said, "il n 'exist pas." So disappeared one of my favorite Paris haunts.

In the evening we sometimes went to the opera or to the theater. "December 26th. We saw Faust. It was very well done. There was a scene where the devil appeared in a pillar. February 6th. At the Odean, we saw The Tempest. It was not so good. Shakespeare wrote it, but it was in French." Bump's diary notes about the trips we took on weekends to the various places around Paris almost invariably began with "We went to ..... in the new Ford." That car was certainly the most useful one we ever had, and gave the boys more pride and pleasure than anything else, for it would pass most of the cars that we met in climbing hills, and all except the racing cars like the Alpha Romeos on ordinary roads. We were in Europe for six months and never took a train or bus to the many parts of the countries we visited.

During that winter and spring, aside from the cathedral towns, we traveled through the chateau country on the Loire and had some delightful experiences at the little inns and auberges where we stayed overnight. One of these I remember well: we had a very good dinner and a wine which the lady proprietor had taken me to the "cave" to select, then a good night's sleep. The next morning, Sunday, we started for Chenanceau, a remarkable chateau built on a bridge over the Loire. On our way we were halted by a guardrail across the railroad track. We waited for fifteen minutes without seeing any sign or sound of an approaching train. So I went into the little station and saw the facteur sitting in a chair with his feet on the desk. When I asked him when the train was due and told him that we had been waiting more than fifteen minutes, he put down his feet, grabbed a timetable and then threw up his hands with the remark, "Oh mon Dieu! C'est domage, c'est Dimanche."

On April 20th we said goodbye to the Merciers and started on our grand tour. As a parting present, Charles Mercier gave us a pewter stein that had been given to him by his uncle, Cardinal Mercier. The Cardinal had won it, as a young student in a debate at the University of Louvain. Ever since then this has been the prize piece in our pewter collection, and a very happy reminder of our stay at the Merciers.

We planned to travel through the south of France to Spain. The first day we went, "in the new Ford" to Vesseley. This was the fourth time that we had visited this charming little town with its unique old abbey built in the tenth century. We had planned to stay there a day, but we liked the place so much, and the Hotel Lion d'Or, a wee bit of an inn where they charged us $10.00 a day for all five of us - two rooms, meals and a garage, that we stayed a week. The abbey was a most fascinating one. It had been in the country that had been conquered by the Huguenots who, in the 15th century, had gone through the Catholic churches and destroyed the statuary and carvings. About 1860 Violet le Duc, a famous French authority on church architecture, discovered that all the capitals on the pillars in the Vesseley abbey were covered with plaster of Paris. He had this carefully removed and the interesting Bible stories carved on these capitals were revealed. When these were first carved in the abbey very few people could read, and their knowledge of the Bible stories was gained from these capitals. One of these that I was showing the kids portrayed a man tearing the jaws of a lion apart; I told them it was Samson. The guardian who was showing us around said, "No, monsieur, that is David, for he has no long hair," and of course he was right.

I had purchased watercolors and drawing paper before we left Paris, and Bumps and I were trying our hands at drawing and painting. He had done some remarkably good ones of racing cars, with models that began to appear in our American makes twenty years later. In his diary he tells of our attempts at pictures of the St. Pierre bridge near Vesseley. He goes on to say, "May 3rd. We left Vesseley in the new Ford and went to Sieulieu where we stopped for lunch. It was the most wonderful dinner we ever ate; everything was perfect, even Dad liked the spinach."

I must go back a bit to tell why we stopped at the little Hotel Briston in Sieulieu for lunch. While we were in Paris, President Nicholas Murray Butler [1] had arrived from Rome where he had been received by his friend, the Pope, and by Mussolini. Dr. and Mrs. Butler asked Mary and I to dine with them at their hotel. That proved to be a very interesting evening, for among other things, he told us of the meal they had had at Sieulieu, and said that if we were going through Dijon and Lyons, we should be sure to stop at the Hotel Briston in that little town, for they served the best food in France. What he said was certainly true, for although we had been in many restaurants in Paris and in the neighboring towns, we had not tasted such food. As a matter of fact, it took us a day to get over the effects of the many rare dishes that they served us.

That same evening Dr. Butler told us so many interesting stories about his stay in Rome. He said that he had been very disturbed about the way the Vatican Library was kept, the fire hazard for the priceless books on wooden shelves and the fact that they kept no card catalogue system. His friend, the Pope, had been the librarian of the Vatican for several years as a cardinal before he was made Pope. Dr. Butler said that the idea occurred to him that if he could persuade the Pope to agree to an exchange of young librarians, it might solve the problem. He suggested this to the Pope and he agreed to receive four librarians, one each from the Library of Congress, Columbia, Harvard and Chicago Universities, and he would send four of his librarians from the Vatican to study in the American libraries.

When the Vatican librarians arrived from Rome, they were given every attention in the above mentioned libraries, but were especially indoctrinated in the Library Bureau card catalogue and filing system. When they returned to the Vatican they could not say enough good things about the American system, and soon the request for further information on that subject arrived. Dr. Butler was the President of the Carnegie Foundation for Peace, and he arranged to send the Vatican a full set of Library bureau files and cards and, more important, a complete set of metal shelves to house the entire Vatican Library as presents to the Vatican. I shall have more to say about that library later on in this story.

That evening, among other things, I asked Dr. Butler who, of all the famous men of intellect and fame that he had known, had the greatest brain and intelligence. Without a moment's hesitation he said, "There is no question about that; the greatest mind that I have ever known is the General of the Order of Jesus, the Jesuit Order. He is little known, for he is always kept in the background, but I have never met a man like him. He is a Polish Jesuit."

The next day, Sunday, we spent in Beaune, a little town in the Burgundy wine country. There we saw a hospital that had been built in 1447, during the Black Plague, by the Court Jester, who had recovered from the epidemic and had vowed he would build a hospital if he were spared. I spent the morning as an American visiting physician and saw a most interesting place. Some of the wards were the same as when the hospital was built, with large beds built into the walls and with brass basins and ewers as old as the wards, but thin from the years of polishing them. The sisters who were the nurses were giving the patients the care that only devoted nuns can give, and the potage they were serving the sick was delicious, for they gave me a portion of it. The library was an art gallery in itself, for there were murals and paintings done by the great artists of the 15th century. I remember one, the Judgment Day, where the artist had given full vent to the portrayal of the most hideous devils shoveling the wicked into the flames and the angels rescuing others and putting them on the way to the pearly gates. "L'Enfer" was quite a painting. The hospital was and had been supported from the income of the vineyards that the Jester had bequeathed when the hospital was built. L'Hospice de Beaune is a famous red burgundy that one can get occasionally in this country, and is one of the finest of the vintages of that famous district.

Bumps' diary shows that we went through Lyons, Albi and Carcassone. His remarks about the last..."We went to Carcassone from Albi, in the new Ford. Carcassone is an old, fortified city with walls all around the place. The town is very old; the streets narrow with a lot of souvenir shops. Carcassone is a failure, I think." And it certainly was, entirely too touristy, and to be admired, should be seen only from a distance.

On May 7th we entered Spain and traveled late until we reached Barcelona. It took some time to find a hotel, and it was 9:30 when I went to the desk and asked if there was a chance of our getting dinner. "Si, Signor, if you will wait a few minutes. Dinner is being served at 10 o'clock." It was a dinner worth waiting for, with delicious Spanish dishes and luscious fruit.

From Barcelona we followed the Mediterranean coast back into France. The diary says, "We left B. in the new Ford. Nothing particular happened. More Ford trucks in Spain. Mum and Sis have the pink eye. May 10th after a night in Montpellier we left in the new Ford and reached St. Raphael. Mum not so well, so we are staying here a few days. May 12th after a beautiful ride, the most wonderful yet, we came through Cannes, Nice and Monte Carlo and arrived on the Italian border. The only thing we had to throw out were the bananas."

The trip through Italy was, in many ways, the most interesting part of our journey. From the border we went to Genoa, where, in passing through one of the main streets, we had a puncture. While the boys were changing the tire, a large crowd gathered and seemed amused at the boys' efforts to put on the new rim. This seemed to annoy Bill, so when they had finished the job, he took off his beret and began passing it through the crowd for contributions, doing so with a perfectly straight face. The crowd rapidly disappeared.

From Genoa to Pisa, to Florence. There we spent a delightful week at the Grand Hotel Aurora, in Fiesole, overlooking Florence from the North of the city. This really was nothing more than a nice pension, but it had a terrace where we had our meals and at night, at dinner after nine o'clock, as the lights began coming over the city, it was a wonderful sight.

Of course the rare art galleries and museums and the matchless buildings of the Renaissance made trips to the city memorable. It was there that we saw and heard Il Duce in one of his state visits to Florence. If there ever were a proud pouter pigeon, it was Mussolini as he rode through the long lanes of plumed soldiers on a black charger, trying to outdo Napoleon in pomposity.

From Florence we drove through the hill towns, Orvietto, Vienna and Assizi. In Assizi we spent three days, for Easter was being observed in that town when we were there. The unique three churches, one above the other, with the famous Giotto paintings and murals on the walls of the middle church and the wonderful singing of the monks and the solemn Easter service made a lasting impression on all of us. The spirit of St. Francis pervades the entire town of Assizi and makes it a place set apart in all of Italy.

When we reached Rome we were a tired and dusty family, but hot baths in our old favorite Hotel Russie made us new. We had two rooms overlooking the church and the little statues that mum and I had seen and liked in 1925. We took many pictures of these again. We wanted the kids to see as many of the famous places in Rome as our stay in that city would permit: St. Peter's, where we saw the Pope at one of the services, the Forum, the Catacombs, the Colliseum and the Vatican, as well as many other wonderful sights including the amazing fountains which are so characteristic of the Eternal City. One can spend months in Rome without exhausting its endless treasures. I shall have more to say about Rome later on.

Our stay in Venice was even more interesting to the kids. We had a porch in a hotel overlooking the Grand Canal and spent a good deal of time in gondolas on the Canal and its tributaries. Of course we saw the Piazza San Marco with its hundreds of pigeons, the Doges Palace, and went to the glass and lace factories and to the Lido. We bought a complete set of Venetian glass and had it shipped to Wilton, but not much of the frail glass in a delicate shade of green is left.

After crossing to the mainland, we resumed our travels "in the new Ford." We drove into the Dolomites where we were unable to resist using our set of pastels; two of the scenes of these mountains and valleys can still be seen in Sis's and Richard's bedrooms. I remember one picnic that we had in a lovely valley, surrounded by high peaks and with a sparkling little river running through the valley below us. It was there that Bill lost one of his sneakers, and I, my prized pipe that I had lost in the Dolomites in 1925. But as before, I found it again, or rather Bill did. The high stark peaks, the wooded valleys and the small emerald lakes make the Dolomites unique, and because they are not so well known to tourists in general, the hotels and inns are unspoiled.

Through Innsbruck we went into Bavaria to Munich where we spent a very happy and restful week in the pension Molsen Husting. Bumps' diary is very largely taken up with the hours that he and Bill spent in their favorite haunt, the Deutches Museum. There they were allowed to work the models of all kinds of machinery and saw models of mines and factories. I am sure they never had a more interesting week during the entire trip. We celebrated Sis's birthday and gave her a fine Zeiss camera.

From Munich we took trips to Nuremberg and to the very old, unspoiled town of Rottenberg, where they were having a fete with everyone dressed in the costumes of centuries ago. On June 13th we drove to the famous little village of Oberammergau, where they were preparing for the presentation of the passion play, given every ten years as a token of the old town's escape from the Black Plague. We stayed in the house of Dominicus Mayer, one of the principal actors. "June 15th, we saw the Passion Play. It lived up to all our hopes, being very real, beautiful and perfectly done." That is a very terse, but significant description of the Play. Mum and I had been concerned about how the kids would take this very realistic portrayal of the Passion Week, which we had read to them from the Gospels. But they and we were profoundly impressed and moved by it. It was not only the superb performance of the Play, but the spirit in which it was done, as well as the tradition of the villagers and the very beautiful setting that made the Play so lastingly impressive.

We then drove to Switzerland through the Rhone valley where we spent the night in a hotel near the Rhone glacier. At two o'clock the next morning, Mary and I wakened just as the sun was touching the top of Mont Blanc. We awakened the children and the five of us watched a most wonderful sunrise over the highest peak in the Alps. It was a thrilling experience for all of us. The next day we had to climb several high passes, one of them the Grinsell, with snow walls eighteen feet high. Bumps remarked in his diary that these steep grades made the Ford boil for the first time. This trip brought us to Interlaken and from there, to high Murren; to get there we had to leave the car and take the funnicular to the little Swiss village, high on the mountain opposite the Jungfrau. Here we spent three most carefree days. But we all tried to do too much walking in the rare atmosphere, and the second day we were all exhausted. On the third day Bill and I went to the Jungfrau and were carried up to the inn near the top in a wee cogwheel train. There we saw people skiing on the snow-covered slopes.

Through Berne and Freiburg we came to the Black Forest, and from there to Strassburg, where, on the 23rd we celebrated Bill's 13th birthday. Then to Paris, stopping at the Hotel Nice for three days. This gave us time to finish packing the things we had left at the Merciers and get our money changed to British currency, as well as for the boys to visit some of their favorite automobile show windows on the Champs Elysees. We then drove back to Bolougne, where we left the Ford in storage and took the channel boat to Folkstone. There we boarded the first train that we had been in since leaving New York, and it took us to London.

In London we stayed at the Thackery Hotel opposite the British Museum. This was a rather rundown temperance affair, but we made up for it by having more than one good dinner at Simpsons. I had to stay in London for a few days to attend the meeting of the Society of Clinical Surgery, so mum and the kids took a train to St. Ives on the Cornwall coast. There they had swimming and sailing between rainy days, which seemed to be common. When I arrived, we went to a little hotel, The Links, situated on the edge of the Laland Golf Course. There the boys and I had great fun playing golf every day for two weeks. Bill made very good friends with two Englishmen who admired his game and played with him on several occasions. We have a dear picture of Bill in his beret with a happy smile, taken during one of the games he played with his British friends.

Mum and Sis took a bus trip through the Lake Country. The boys and I met them later in Wilton, England. There we bought the Welsh dresser and the walnut chest that have decorated our various homes ever since. We then went to Edinburgh, and from there, to St. Andrews where the boys and I had the best week of golf ever. The Old Course and Edens were tried on different days and in different weather and were very different depending upon the wind and the Scotch mist. When I was in Edinburgh, I met Bill Herrick, one of the medical attendings at the Medical Center. He was a fine golfer and was on his way to St. Andrews. So when we arrived he and I had more than one good time on the Old Course. The St. Andrews caddies were old professionals and knew the course and its vagaries - the traps were all named - like a book. If you did not take their advice as to the club to use or the direction to take, disaster was sure.

One day Bill Herrick had a short, sawed off caddie named Sandy MacPherson. For the first five holes Bill made splendid shots, which were commended by Sandy with quotations from Robby Burns [2]. On the sixth tee Bill sliced his drive into the winnies toward the sea. Sandy said nothing and put down another ball on the tee for Bill, which he drove straight and far. As we walked off the tee, Bill said to Sandy, "You didn't quote any Robby Burns after I sliced that ball." Sandy winked at him and said, "Aye, I dinna, but I coulda."

Sunday at St. Andrews was a very Scotch Presbyterian day - no golf or any other form of amusement. I was taken to task for doing a little watercolor on the links. We went to the old Kirk and, on coming out, walked through the old graveyard. Many of the headstones were marked "Property of so-and-so." One tall one caught our eye. It was the headstone of the grave of a former golf champion of Scotland. On the stone were two crossed golf sticks, and below them was the phrase, "Far and True."

We returned to Edinburgh and traveled to the east coast to take a boat to the Isle of Skye. This was a typical highland spot, the home of the MacLeans and the MacDonalds. Uncle William MacLean, aunt Maggie's husband had come to this country from that island. Most of the people spoke Gaelic and many of them had bushy red hair and beards, looking very much like their Heeland cattle. The days alternated between dense fog and the most brilliant sunshine. The streams coming down from the mountains were fishermen's dreams, for they were the home of trout and salmon.

On our way back to Edinburgh mum got a fine plaid cape and I bought two bolts of Scotch tweed which I later had made into two sport jackets, one of which is a tan color, mum's favorite, and which is still as good as ever.

Our last day in Edinburgh gave us a chance to see many of the famous buildings and I was able to revisit the Royal Infirmary, the home of so many of the great medical figures of the Edinburgh School. After returning to London on the Flying Scot, we took the train to the channel and the boat to Bologne. There we picked up the Ford and sailed back to New York on the old Minnekahda, then back to Wilton. Thus ended the Red Letter Year for our family, for it was the most interesting one of our lives, one that has meant so much to all of us in so many ways.

Footnotes

1. **Nicholas Murray Butler (1862-1947)**

    An American philosopher and educator who had studied at Paris and Berlin. He became the President of Columbia University in 1902. An advocate of peace through education, Butler helped to establish the Carnegie Endowment for International Peace. He was a 1931 Nobel Peace Prize Laureate.

2. **Robert Burns (1759-1796)**

    Also known as the "Poet of Scotland". Robert Burns achieved immortality through his efforts to reinvigorate the Scottish vernacular through his poetry and his rescue of hundreds of the folk songs of Scotland.

Chapter Twelve

A tragedy and more Europe

1930 - 1937

On our return there was much to be done in catching up with the doings of the months that we had been away. I found that things had gone well in the surgical department during my absence due to the unselfish work of Hugh and John. It almost made me feel that I was a good executive, having picked such able associates. We had able residents and the training program was functioning smoothly.

The question about the schools for the children was one of immediate importance. Sis had been accepted in Radcliffe, Bumps was returning to Eaglebrook and we had entered Bill there. That fall they left us to continue their studies. We moved to the house on Fieldstone Road, and mum soon showed again her genius in making it a most attractive home. That was the beginning of our happy associations with the Riverdale and Fieldstone people. Mum started the first Thrift Shop in the community, which she managed so successfully for the next nine years, very much to the benefit of the Riverdale Association and the low-income people in that area.

In January of 1933 I had to go to Puerto Rice to lecture at the School of Tropical Disease that, with the University Hospital, was affiliated with Columbia University. For ten days I was kept busy lecturing and visiting other hospitals on the island, as well as meeting many of the doctors working there. The depression was on and I left as soon as I could, flying back to the States. In 1930 I had accepted renewal of an offer to go on full-time, so that the question of getting an income from practice was not a problem. Learning how to curtail expense was, for I found that the family income had decreased by about fifty per cent. But that is what one has to expect if he works on a full-time basis.

When I returned to Fieldstone I found that Bill had gone on a ski trip to the Adirondacks as a member of the Eaglebrook team. He sent us a picture of the team in which he appeared to be in the finest form, heavier and stronger than ever. His letter from Lake Placid was most enthusiastic and full of his plans for coming for the Easter vacation.

On March 27th, 1933, Bill came to Fieldstone from Eaglebrook and met me on the steps of the house as I drove in from the hospital. He looked so well and handsome. The next day he and mum and Eunie went to Wilton, Bill's favorite place of all others. That evening Mary and Eunie returned to Fieldstone. The next morning, after a hearty breakfast, Bill and his friend Henry took one of the old Fords on a ride over one of the less frequented roads leading to Norwalk. It had rained hard the day before, causing washouts on some of the roads. Something went wrong with the car when it struck a hole at the bottom of a bridge. The car turned over, the side of it falling on Bill's abdomen. People nearby saw the accident and called the ambulance from the Norwalk Hospital. When Bill arrived there, the surgeon whom I knew, examined Bill and called me at the Presbyterian immediately and told me that Bill was seriously injured, advising me to come to Norwalk as soon as possible. I left at once and reached the Norwalk Hospital regardless of speed limits. When I saw Bill he had had a hypodermic, but was conscious and assured me that the accident was nobody's fault.

The drive back to New York with Bill in the ambulance, his condition growing rapidly worse, was a tragic experience for me. I had telephoned Johnnie St. John before leaving Norwalk so that, when we arrived at the Medical Center, John and Barclay Parsons had everything ready. They took Bill to the operating room immediately and he was given blood transfusions until his shock condition was improved enough to begin the operation. Mum, Sis and Eunie had come to the hospital. I went in to see

Bill before the anesthesia was started and said, "Bill, keep the chin up." He smiled and said, "I will, Dad." As a family we waited near the operating room with good friends with us. But when John came out from the operating room to speak to me, I could tell from his drawn expression that there was little hope for dear Bill. That evening at eleven o'clock he died peacefully without regaining consciousness. When we learned what his injuries were, aside from the abdominal condition, for he had a fractured spine as well, we could not have wished for a different outcome.

So came the first tragedy in our family - a sudden and shocking loss. Bill was in the prime of his young manhood; tall, strong, and so handsome, as dear and lovable a lad as ever lived. He was always generous, outgiving, and so devoted to all of us in the family. His keen sense of humor and delightful chuckle and contagious laugh when he heard a good story, or saw something really funny, was unforgettable. He loved the early morning and the outdoors, especially as he saw them in Wilton and Nantucket. What a dear lad he was!

That next summer we decided to go abroad again and planned to spend several weeks in Vienna. The four of us sailed from New York, landing at Le Havre on the 9th of July, and from there we went to Paris where we spent two days visiting our old haunts. Early the next morning we drove through silent streets to the airport and took a plane to Vienna, passing through Strassburg, Nuremberg and Prague. In Nuremberg we got the first impression of the Nazi regime in the soldiers and police that were very prominent. Just after we had started to leave the airfield the engine caught fire and we had to return to where we had started. After they had extinguished the fire, the flight was continued. The plane was an old one and looked as if the wings were held together with huge safety pins. That we ever landed safely in Vienna was a miracle. Bumps had an unfortunate experience in having his raincoat showered by a fat German who became violently air sick. His baggage was sent by mistake to Romania, too, and was delayed in its recovery for several days.

We found a pension run by Frau Hursells and her daughter; it proved convenient, but not too comfortable. We had German lessons from the fraulein in the mornings without too much effect. In fact we did not feel energetic for much in Vienna. There was a saying in Vienna, "Everything in Vienna is critical, but not serious." Every one in that city seemed not to take life too seriously, but with plenty of "gemutlichkeit". After the First World War the city was the epitome of depleted Austria. Everything was shabby and there were many sad-looking beggars to be seen in all parts of the city - women holding little children with their hands out for whatever coins they could get. One of the things that I saw was very typical of the saying that nothing was serious: one saw men playing chess everywhere and at all times; a newspaper vendor calling out his papers while intently playing the game, and not pleased to be interrupted by someone wanting to buy a paper. Another characteristic finding was our hearing string quartets, especially in the residential parts of the city and in the suburbs.

During the first month we were there I rented a cello and applied to the music conservatory for a room where I could practice. The very genial soul who was in charge of the rooms said that there were very few people using the rooms in the summer, and that I was welcome to any room that I chose; he refused any money for the rental. My practice was desultory and I did not do justice to the generosity of the man who gave me the room.

We met Dr. Adler in the city, among other doctors there, and were asked one Sunday to attend a tea at Dr. Adler's home in the country. Bumps' comment in his diary, which he again kept on our European trip, reads, "Went to Adler's country place for the afternoon with a lot of queer ducks." Many of our evenings were spent in the park listening to endless Strauss waltzes, with which we got fed up, or else we went to the coller suburbs or to the Wienerwald.

Bumps and I decided that we needed more exercise, so we took a plane for Salzburg and spent three days listening to the Mozart festival and seeing the interesting play, Jederman, which was given outdoors on the Salzburg Plaza. We then rented bicycles and started to travel through the Salzkammergud country. But we soon found that it was mostly mountains, and by the time we had gone fifty kilometers, walking most of the way because of the steep hills, we asked a Tyrolean how far it was to Bad Ausee. His reply was, "About two pipes," meaning the time that it would take to smoke the long and large-bowled Tyrolean pipes. After another long period of hill climbing and pushing of bicycles, we reached the charming town and engaged a room on the second story overlooking a beautiful lake. The long hill hikes had worn out the soles of my shoes, so that I had to sit on the porch in my stocking feet while my only pair of shoes was being re-soled. Bumps, in the meantime, had secured a fishing license and had spent the day fishing on the lake, with what success I do not remember. The cost of our room and meals came to about three dollars for both of us! We had a long rest in this beautiful spot on the lake where the famous Viennese surgeon of the previous century, Billroth, had his summer home. I had an engraving of Billroth, standing on his porch, which I gave to the surgical department when I retired.

But we decided that the idea of bicycling further was a poor one, so we put our wheels on a bus and came back to Salzburg. There we met mum and Sis, and the next few days took a train back to Vienna, much to everyone's regret for it was a dusty, hot ride as compared to the flight by plane.

After another week in Vienna Bumps and I got tickets on the Europa to return to New York because he had to make up work that he had missed at school. Mum and Sis came later on a French boat. Bumps and I left on the 15th of August for Berlin and Bremen, taking a third class car, much to our regret, for it proved to be a hot and utterly stupid train trip. A hot bath at the hotel in Berlin and a very good dinner that evening restored our humor and prepared us to see the funny and stilted side of the Nazi regime that was evident all about us. The only part of the ocean voyage that I remember was the dreadful vibration, day and night, in the stern part of the ship where the service of the waiters and stewards was inexcusably bad and discourteous. They certainly showed no love for Americans.

Chapter Thirteen

Mother's death and the Scandinavian trip

1937

In the summer of 1937 the Society of Clinical Surgery had decided to take a foreign trip to the Scandinavian countries. As President of the Society at that time, it was my duty to go with the members who had signed to attend the meeting. We had planned to take the Swedish ship Gripsholm in the latter part of June. The night before we were to sail I had a long distance call from Eunice saying that mother had developed an intestinal obstruction and was in need of surgery. I told her that I would take a plane to Chicago and from there to Fish Creek where mother had been spending the summer with the Clarks. A very good surgeon from Milwaukee I knew, was near Fish Creek at the time, and I told Eunice to get him to operate immediately; that I would come at once.

The next morning I took the first plane to Chicago and then a private one to Fish Creek so that I arrived there in the afternoon, after mother had been operated upon. She was in the hospital in Sturgeon Bay, near Fish Creek, and was her courageous self when I came in to see her. The surgeon had explored her under local anesthesia, but found an inoperable condition. She apparently realized this, for she said, "I know they have done all that could be done." The next morning when Eunice and I came to see her she said, "It is time for me to go. I have had a wonderfully full life and have lived to a ripe old age (87). I want to have you and the girls meet me here for a family reunion." Mary Barton had flown from Shreveport, arriving a short time before I did. We came to her

119

bedside. She said, "While I am still competent mentally, I want to give you messages for you and your grandchildren." This she did, and then she said, "I would like to have a little service. It has always seemed a pity that a funeral service should be held when one is dead and can take no part in it." Mother then asked me to read the 13th Chapter of Corinthians I, the 91st Psalm and the 23rd. Then she said, "All three of you have good voices and I would like you to sing 'Abide with me' and 'Rock of Ages', two of my favorite hymns." I said, "Mother, that will be hard for us." She said, "I know that, but I expect you to do it for me." We did just that, and then she said a beautiful prayer for all of us and her dear ones. After this, she turned to me and said, "It is time for me to go to sleep. It isn't necessary for me to wake again, is it?" With this, she closed her eyes and after that she slept peacefully for the next thirty-six hours, with the help of a sedative and died without regaining consciousness. Later Robert and Eunice had a headstone placed over her grave, with her name, "wife of the Reverend William L. Whipple, missionaries to Persia," and, below this, "Go ye into all the world and preach the Gospel." So ended a wonderful life, the most unselfish that I have ever known, and which left a memory that will always be a benediction.

From Terre Haute I took a plane to New York, and two days later, the Queen Mary to Southampton, then to London and, from there, a plane to Copenhagen, where I joined the Society group. But on the Queen Mary I had contracted a cold, which was not improved on the plane to Copenhagen, and a sinus condition stayed with me the rest of the trip. We went to Stockholm for several days, and had an interesting time at the surgical clinics in that city, as well as seeing the sights and scenery of the cleanest city in Europe. One sees there the finest taste in modern architecture and furnishings; the City Hall being one of the best examples of the modern trend in building.

The Society was invited to a luncheon at the country home of the Professor of Surgery of the University of Stockholm. He had married the niece of Nobel, the very wealthy founder of the Nobel Prizes. She had inherited a fortune, but, in her own right, was a most talented and remarkable woman. Mother of five sons and three daughters (the most beautiful of the women that we saw in Sweden and there were many such beauties in that country), she was an accomplished landscape painter, a mountain climber, and she wove the most remarkable tweed cloth that was as fine as any to be found in Scotland. This she made from the wool of their sheep on their estate. All of her five sons were wearing suits made from the cloth, which she had woven.

The luncheon at the long table, seating more than thirty people, was an elaborate affair, preceded by a smorgasbord. The table decorations were unusual; they consisted of many varieties of nasturtiums and ivy hanging from a series of glass globes above the table. All the "skaaling" was done with French champagne, and everyone was "skaaled", so you can imagine how gay the party became before the ceremonies were over. As President of the Society, I had to respond to more than one of the host's speeches, and I kept this in mind through the "skaaling". But what a party that was! One of the first things I did when we returned to the city was to buy a set of these globes in different sizes, and they were unusual decorations in our living room in different houses for many years.

From Stockholm we went to Oslo and sailed through some of the Norwegian fjords. The Society then went to London, some of them going on to Scotland, but I came back to New York. One of the interesting reactions we got in Scandinavia was the real dread those countries had of the threat of the Nazis. They seemed to be more aware of the things that were impending than the rest of the world.

Chapter Fourteen

Pancreatic surgery

1933 - 1946

My work in the surgery of the biliary tract and the spleen had been increasing rapidly, and I had to delegate more and more of it to some of my younger associates and residents who had worked with me in those fields. The surgery of the pancreas had been more or less an unexplored field so far as the tumors of that organ were concerned. The very recent recognition of tumors of the islet cells of the pancreas, which gave a clinical picture identical with that caused by an overdose of insulin - for these symptoms were caused by an overproduction of insulin by the islet cells of these tumors - had intrigued me greatly. In 1933 I began to get such patients from the Neurological Institute in the Medical Center where they had been sent because of their nervous disorders. The first such patient whom I operated upon made such an immediate, brilliant recovery that I was assigned at once any others that came to the Institute, and within the year I had equally good results with five more such patients. The study of their pre-operative symptoms, and especially their fasting blood sugar findings, gave a clear cut diagnostic picture. When I first published these findings in the *International Journal of Surgery* calling attention to the three essential signs for the diagnosis of islet cell tumors, it attracted immediate attention and ever since then has been called "The Whipple Triad". Before retiring from the Presbyterian I had operated on 39 such cases, finding a tumor, or tumors, in 35. At that time this was the largest series of such operated patients in the surgical literature.

In 1935 we began work on the more serious cancers of the pancreas, which in the past had been considered inoperable. I had operated upon a woman with such a tumor, using catgut for the suture and ligature material. The patient, died two days later, and the autopsy showed that the catgut had been digested and absorbed by the digestive juices of the pancreas resulting in leakage and peritonitis. My senior resident, Hap Mullins, discussed these findings with me and asked me why I did not use silk technique that had been so successful in our islet cell tumors. This appealed to me immediately, and when the next patient came with a cancer of the pancreas, assigned to Barclay Parson's service, I assisted him with Mullins in a radical operation. The patient made a good recovery. We reported this operation at the next meeting of the American Surgical Association [1], which attracted immediate attention, for this was the first successful operation that had been attempted in this country. Previous attempts by a few French and German surgeons had been given up as prohibitive.

This started us on a new field of radical cancer surgery. The first few patients we operated on were done in two stages because of the presence of deep jaundice in too many of them. But in 1940, with the discovery of vitamin K by a Danish physiologist [2], a vitamin that prevented bleeding in jaundiced patients, I was able to do the first one-stage radical operation for the removal of the head of the pancreas and the entire duodenum. That patient did very well and since then the one-stage operation has become the operation chosen by surgeons in this country and abroad. Some of these tumors give better late results than others, depending upon the location of the cancer and its type. At best, it is one of the most serious kinds of malignant disease, and more recently some surgeons have removed the entire pancreas with results that have still to be evaluated.

These eleven years, from 1935 to 1946, were the most active and productive years of my life as a surgeon, for we were dealing with new and original fields and I had a fine team to work with, both as attendings and residents, with very adequate laboratory facilities and a great deal of clinical material which the reports from the surgical service had brought to the hospital. During this time we had originated the so-called porto-caval shunt operation used in bypassing the blood from the portal venous system of the gastro-intestinal tract and spleen to the inferior vena cava, bringing blood from the lower extremities and abdominal wall. This was used in patients with cirrhosis, or where portal blood was obstructed. We started this work with Pete Rousselot and Arthur Blakemore [3] and before I retired we had done some sixty of these operations; Rousselot did several hundred of them. Now these operations are being done in all the leading surgical clinics.

Footnotes

1. Whipple AO, Parsons WB, Mullins CR. Treatment of Carcinoma of the Ampulla of Voter. *Ann Surg* 1935; 102: 763-79.

2. **Henrik Dam (1895-1976)**

    A Danish chemist known for his studies of the metabolism of sterols and the discovery of vitamin K. During WWII he sojourned in North America, receiving in 1943 the Nobel Prize for physiology and medicine. He returned to Denmark in 1946.

3. **Arthur H. Blakemore (1897-1970)**

    A graduate of Johns Hopkins School of Medicine (1922) who joined the surgical staff at Columbia-Presbyterian Medical Center (1928). He pioneered the development of synthetic material for vascular surgery and is best known for perfecting a balloon tamponade of esophageal varices in 1954 (Segstaken-Balkemore Tube).

Chapter Fifteen

Operation in Rome, the Pope and Europe

1941

Because of this experience I was kept busy in reading papers at surgical societies and clinical meetings. At the 1939 meeting of the American Surgical Association, as President of the Association, I had to read the Presidential Address and chose as my subject, "Wound Healing," a topic that had always interested me. This meeting was held in St. Louis, where Mary and I were the guests of the Grahams. Evarts was the Professor of Surgery there for thirty-four years, a record, and Helen was Professor of Pharmacology.

In 1938 I operated upon Mr. Myron Taylor [1], who later was appointed the ambassador to the Vatican. He made a good recovery and I got to know him and his wife well. They had a fine house in the city and a big estate on Long Island, to which Mary and I were invited on more than one occasion. One morning at two o'clock, during the latter part of June, 1941, I was awakened by the phone by Mrs. Taylor who said that she had just received a cable from Florence telling of Mr. Taylor's serious condition with jaundice and a severe gastric hemorrhage, with what the doctors in Florence had diagnosed recurrent gall-stones. They urged her to go to Florence immediately. It was obvious that she was dreadfully worried and anxious. She asked me if I would be willing to fly to Italy with her and to be prepared to do any surgery that might be indicated. This was quite a decision to have to make on the spur of the moment, so I told Mary what the message was, and asked what she thought I should do.

Like the great help she always was, she said that I had operated on Mr. Taylor and knew what the findings were; that it was up to me to go and be of any help I could be to him. So I replied to Mrs. Taylor that I would come with her and would bring a special nurse and instruments if surgery were necessary. The next morning I flew to Washington, and because Mr. Taylor was the Roosevelt representative at the Vatican, we were given diplomatic passports at once.

The next day we took a plane to Lisbon, and had to stay there two days until we could get a plane to Rome from Barcelona. The night we spent in Barcelona at the Ritz Hotel, which was once the swankiest in Spain. Then it was anything but that, because Spain had just had a revolution and parts of the city had been badly bombed. The food was hardly edible and there was no service. We saw chicken coops on the rooftops of some of the houses, for eggs were not to be had in the markets.

The following morning we took an Italian plane for Rome, but we had to land on the scorching airfield in Sardinia because of the British planes that had been sighted near that island. Since Italy was at war with England we would have been sitting ducks for the British Spitfires had they seen an Italian plane. That dreadfully hot afternoon in the sordid, suffocating airport office, with Mrs. Taylor frantic because of the news she had received just as we were leaving Barcelona saying that Mr. Taylor was much worse, was as trying a six hours as I have ever spent anywhere.

We landed on the airport in Rome just as the French delegation had arrived to receive the conditions of surrender to the Italians. I never saw a more dejected lot of Frenchmen as those officers were, nor a more arrogant and pompous lot of Italian officers that met the Frenchmen at the airport.

We soon boarded another plane for Florence, due to the good offices of my friend Rafael Bastienelli who had been called from Rome to Florence as a consultant in Mr. Taylor's case. When we arrived at the beautiful Taylor villa, not far below Fiesole, I found the patient in critical condition, the result of the combination of severe loss of blood and deep jaundice. He was in great need of blood transfusion. The Florence doctors said that they had given him 200cc and were horrified when I told them that he needed at least 2000cc more.

The housekeeper of the villa was the wife of a police officer in Florence and through her I soon had five husky policemen, redolent with garlic but with high hemoglobins. After matching their blood types with that of the patient we had three strong donors. From one of them I gave a liter of blood to Mr. Taylor that evening; and another the next morning. Thanks to the good offices and understanding of Bastienelli, of whom I have spoken in our trip in 1925, we decided to take the patient to the Bastienelli Clinic in Rome the next afternoon since Mr. Taylor had improved following the transfusions. A private car was engaged with a comfortable bed in it. The question of how to get him from the villa to the train was answered by an ambulance. I had heard that they had an ambulance in Florence, but when I had seen it in 1925, I thought that they were making a movie of it, with the litter bearers in their ancient costumes that were used in the 15th century during the Black Plague.

The housekeeper told me that the ambulance drivers and assistants still had to wear these costumes because the litter bearers had been endowed with the proviso that these costumes would continue to be worn in perpetuity. The ambulance arrived, four men got out of it wearing long black nightgown-like robes and high, peaked hats with two holes for the eyes and a long nose, also black. The housekeeper was able to persuade the four men to take off the hoods before entering the villa, but they insisted on wearing the black robes. I tried to explain things to Mr. Taylor, but he was running a high temperature and was not too clear in his mind. While the four men were carrying him down the three flights of winding stairs and with me at his side, he looked up and said, "Where are the candles?"

We arrived that evening in Rome and had to drive through unlighted streets to the clinic for they were keeping a complete blackout at night during that year of the war. One occasionally heard the policemen yelling "luce" whenever they saw any evidence of a light on in any building. Bastienelli, when he was called in consultation in Florence, realized that Mr. Taylor was in urgent need of surgery, but did not wish to operate until Mrs. Taylor had been notified. When he heard that she and I, as Mr. Taylor's former surgeon, were on their way to Florence, he told me that he was very glad to be out of a difficult situation with the doctors in that city. When we arrived in his clinic he could not have been more helpful and cooperative.

The next morning everything, including the instruments that I had brought with me, was ready. The thing that I was most concerned about was the anesthetic, for I knew nothing about their methods, nor was Bastienelli confident about giving the patient a general anesthetic and urged me to operate under local anesthesia with Novocain, which I had brought with me. This I used, but it was hard on the patient and the surgeon, although much safer. Bastienelli assisted me very skillfully, and helped me no end for the operating nurses spoke no English, which he did very well. He could have made it very difficult for me if he had wanted to, but quite the opposite; he gave me valuable suggestions. We were able to remove the large gallstone that was obstructing the common bile duct, but did not attempt to deal with the duodenal ulcer because the patient had stopped bleeding and we did not want to prolong the operation considering the condition he was in.

Much to our relief, everyone included, Mr. Taylor made a good recovery for the operation, and after the first week, I began to have spare time at my disposal. Of course there was a great deal of publicity connected with the operation and the operator, and for the first week, daily bulletins had to be given to the press, as well as to the Secretary of the Vatican who came every morning to interview me about Mr. Taylor's illness. Mr. Taylor was playing a very important role at the Vatican at that critical period for the Holly See.

Two weeks after the operation I was told that the Pope wished to see me in a private audience, to get first-hand impressions about Mr. Taylor. This was arranged for a Tuesday morning when Mrs. Taylor and I were to meet His Holiness in his private study in the Vatican. This meant that I had to hire a long-tailed dress suit and starched shirtfront and white tie, which were required by protocol for any man having the distinction of a private audience. I was directed to one of the streets near the Vatican where, after trying on the second suit, I found one that fit me perfectly.

On Tuesday morning Mrs. Taylor and I arrived at a special entrance to the Vatican and, after passing through a long line of Swiss guards in their 14th Century picturesque uniforms, we were escorted to the Pope's study by one of his secretaries. After entering the study we were alone with the Holy Father. As we started to kneel before him to kiss his ring he said that the formalities were not necessary, and in very good English he soon made us feel at ease. He immediately wanted to know all about "My dear friend, Myron Taylor." He asked very pertinent and intelligent questions and it was evident that he was glad to get the latest news about his friend's condition and progress. After half an hour with the Pope, he went to his desk and brought out several fine rosaries, which he blessed and asked if we had special Catholic friends to whom we would like to give one of these. I said that I had two devout Catholic friends, our cook, who had given me a St. Andrew's token before taking the plane on this trip, and Charley Cosstello, the man who had been the usher at the entrance to the College of P & S for over forty years and a great favorite of the medical students during that time. The Pope gave two of these a special blessing and said he was glad to send the rosaries to them.

The Pope Pius XII [2] is one of the really few holy men that I have met, very simple in manner, but with the greatest sincerity. He appeared frail and yet with his entire faculties alert, and with the kindest expression and voice that one could ever hear. His remarks about the war and all that it meant to the Church and to God fearing people were very significant. I remember one remark that he made, "This war and all its problems have been, and are, a terrible trial, but this is not the first time that the Church has had to meet such crises, and as in the past, the Church will meet this one." When I returned to New York and gave the rosary to our cook, Canadian Mary, and to Charley Cosstello, they were received with the greatest appreciation, and with tears running down their cheeks. They said they could have nothing that would mean so much to them as the present that I had brought to them directly from the Holy Father.

During the five weeks that I was in Rome I made the morning visit to Mr. Taylor with Professor Bastienelli and later in the afternoon and evening by myself. But I had an increasing amount of spare time on my hands. Mr. Taylor gave me a personal note to Cardinal Tisserant, the librarian of the Vatican, a delightful Turkish scholar and a leading authority in Semitic languages. This letter and the knowledge that I had operated on Mr. Taylor gave me an entree to the Vatican that few others could have had. When I presented my letter to Cardinal Tisserant, he was examining theses that had been submitted by students seeking advanced degrees. They were of a wide variety, all the way from a study of Mexican lilies to a study of one of the earliest chants of the Coptic liturgy. In the course of our conversation I told him that I had studied classical Arabic with Enno Littman at Princeton. The Cardinal had been very polite, but when he heard me mention Littman, he became even more cordial and said that he knew him and had the highest regard for Littman's eminence as one of the world's leading Semitic scholars. This was another open sesame, for the Cardinal conducted me personally to parts of the Vatican Library that I could not have seen otherwise.

One of the most interesting places in the Library was the laboratory where they were studying methods for preserving their very old manuscripts and incunabula. They had developed and were using a method, which consisted of spraying a very thin film of gelatin over the pages, followed by a similar spray of formalin, which fixed the gelatin without affecting the translucency of the writing. This had proven so effective that Pierpont Morgan had sent his oldest and rarest manuscript of the Coptic Bible to be so treated. When it was returned to the Morgan Library he had a facsimile made of it, and sent it to the Vatican, the only copy in the world.

Another unusual and delightful experience occurred during these weeks when I visited so many places that I had heard of, but never seen;

places that I am sure that I shall never see again in that Eternal City. The church of San Clemente had been described as one of the most interesting in Rome. When I went there one afternoon I was met at the front entrance by an old padre who asked me to write my name in the large visitor's book. I did so, and when he read my name, he said, "Why, you are the long-distance surgeon who operated on the American Ambassador to the Vatican. We are very honored to have you visit us." With that he called a younger priest, Brother Ephriam who was an artist, and asked him to act as my guide.

The church had been taken over by the Irish Benedictines some seventy years previously. One of the padres had become very interested in the history and archeology of the church. He discovered that the present building, built in the 14th Century, had been built over an older church. When they had finished excavating the older church they found unique murals on the walls of the church, which had been painted in the 8th Century. Further research revealed the fact that a much older chapel was to be found beneath the 8th Century church. When it was discovered, they found that it had been the home of the fourth Pope, named Clement. He had been a close friend of the disciple Peter, by whom he had been converted to Christianity. Before that he had been a Mithraist, fire worshipper. This excavation revealed not only the home of Clement, but also adjoining it, a small Mithra, or chapel, with a fire altar still intact. All these lowest structures were bordering on the more ancient Sabine wall. All these rare relics were shown to me with enthusiasm by the charming young Irish priest and artist. He was especially ardent in showing me the murals in the second church, and later took me for tea with the other monks.

Being alone and with so much spare time, I was able to see so much more of Rome that I had never seen before as well as those parts of the city with which I was familiar. One of the latter was the Sistine Chapel where I spent an entire morning, alone, in that unique art gallery. During the war with the restrictions on visitors in that city there were so few sightseers that the guides, formerly so numerous, had practically disappeared. I met only one in the Forum while I was making a sketch of the capital of one of the columns. He asked me if I wanted a guide. I said that I was not sightseeing and asked him why he did not offer to guide a group of Germans who were walking through the Forum. He looked at them and with much venom said, "Those Tedeschi need no guide, they are spies. Curse them and their nation!"

The feeling on the part of the Italians toward the Germans, soldiers as well as civilians, who had invaded Rome in great numbers, was very bitter. They had discovered the ruthless and arbitrary ways of the German military who were in control of the city and had to take it, whether they liked it or not. After I accompanied the Taylors back to Florence, I returned to Rome and spent three days in a hotel there where there were a good many German officers. They made a point of coming to the dining room a good half hour after the rest of the people had entered, including the Italian officers. When the German officers came in, the Italian officers had to stand and salute, but on more than one occasion I heard them cursing the Tedeschi, as they called the Germans. There was no enthusiasm for the war in any part of the city or the country, so far as I could learn. The only cheering that could be heard was when it was forced by the presence of Mussolini's henchmen. Formerly one heard singing everywhere, city as well as country. But the whole time that I was in Italy that year I never heard a voice raised in song.

My last week in Rome was taken up largely in trying to get a plane that would take me back to Lisbon, where I hoped to get a plane to America. I had bad luck in getting any mail, having had only two letters the whole time I was away due to the war and the censoring of the mails. I had met Mr. Matthews, a correspondent of the New York Times. He said that if I would arrange to have someone of the family at the Times office in New York, he could manage to have me speak to them after he had finished his message. This I was able to do, and it was a blessed relief to hear Mary's dear voice and to know that they were all well.

I was finally able to get a seat on a plane to Lisbon. During the days that I pestered the Air Offices I had noticed a very distinguished elderly gentleman who came to the Offices as frequently as I. Early one morning

I arrived at the airport before any of the stores were open, and the only things that I could get for lunch (they did not serve any food on the plane), were four small sandwiches and two plums. On entering the plane I saw an empty seat, and after taking it, I discovered to my surprise that sitting next to me was the distinguished gentleman whom I had seen frequently before. I did not introduce myself; in fact, not until we had landed in the airfield in Barcelona with the temperature in the high 90s and found ourselves sitting under the remains of a grape arbor, did I learn that my companion was Captain John A. Gade [3], the Naval Intelligence Officer in Europe, who was then living in Lisbon. I asked him if he would share my poor lunch with me. In his book, *All My Born Days*, he has this to say about our meeting: "It was still dark when the nervous crowd collected in the Alla Littoria's offices - we would have to be late in starting. How long? Surely an hour; possibly three. What is the trouble, I asked. Thanks to the presence of an Embassy servant, I was able to learn that British planes were over the waters we had to fly, and they would naturally try to shoot us down. It would be the irony of fate if I were shot down by the service I had been trying to assist to the best of my ability during the previous days in Switzerland.

"Among the patient waiting crowd was a man one could have singled out anywhere as one of character and mark. He had a firm mouth and chin, a sensitive nose, and above it the eyes of an eagle. I looked at his hands; they were thin and capable and used to work. I felt certain that he was an American. Finally we took off, and a few hours later, came down to a dusty improvised Barcelona airport, the regular one having been destroyed by bombing during the recent civil war. Few of us had thought of bringing our luncheon, so we all made a bolt for the restaurant. However starved our condition, one short look was sufficient to turn our stomachs. Such pathetic scraps of food as were set out on the counter were literally hidden from view by flies; the cheese could have walked off by itself.

"I returned to the blistering sun. Under the shade of a grape arbor, I passed my distinguished American with a very modest luncheon spread out on his lap, scarcely sufficient for one, I thought. 'Didn't you lunch?'

he asked me in a friendly American voice. 'No, it was too filthy; I couldn't stand the looks of it'. 'Well do sit down here', he pushed along the bench, making room, 'and share my lunch.' 'No, thank you,' I answered, 'there is not enough for one.' He insisted in a manner no gentleman could refuse, so I gave my name as I seated myself beside him. He replied, 'My name is Dr. Whipple.'

"I knew then that he was the great surgeon, the Surgical Director of the Medical Center, who had flown over to save the life of Myron Taylor, our Ambassador to the Vatican. I had sized up the man correctly."

I saw Captain Gade on more than one occasion after reaching Lisbon and he gave me very good leads as to where to go to see the worthwhile places in and about that city. When I landed in Lisbon, I had expected to have a reservation at one of the hotels, but when I went there they said that the man who was to have left was ill and they had no vacancies. They gave me the address of a place that they assured me would give me a room. The city was then the bottleneck of Europe, especially for those trying to get out of Germany and the other countries, which were at war. When I arrived at the address that had been given me, I entered what was evidently a tenement house. One look at the room and the bed, which was occupied by fast crawling bedbugs, convinced me that the nearby park was a much better place to spend the night. This I did, but the next morning I returned to the hotel where I had stayed on my way to home, and told them that I would stay in the hotel lobby until they gave me a room. They swore that there was not a room to be had, but by ten o'clock that evening I was given a six by eight room just to one side of the lift on the fourth floor. It had no window, and I had to stay in that cubbyhole for the next week whenever I was not wandering the streets or haunting the air offices. Never was I in a more dreary and loathsome city. It was full of people who were suspicious of everyone else, and there were Germans as well as spies of other nationalities everywhere. The only chance one had of getting the London Times, or any other Allied paper, was to get to the newspaper kiosk before the German spies bought the entire edition. At the table, where good food and wines were served, no one spoke to his neighbor, but cast furtive glances at each other. There was an Australian officer who sat next to me for four days but did not speak to me until he had made certain I was an American.

One morning I was in a hurry to get to the air office and saw an empty taxi in the square. My attempts to give the address in French, German and Italian were feeble. The taxi driver said, "Boss, why don't you talk American?" When I asked him where he had learned it, he said, "I used to live in Nantucket several years." When I told him that that was exactly where I was trying to go, he got very excited, told me his name, and that he was one of three brothers who had been in the antique business. He asked me to be sure to see his brothers, whom I knew, and to tell them that he was well and wished that he could come back to Nantucket.

The morning after I reached the family, who were in Nantucket, I walked out to the golf course and saw three men on the first tee. They asked me if I cared to make up a foursome. They introduced themselves, and two of them were the two brothers to whom I had promised to bring the messages from their brother in Lisbon. This I immediately did, to the utter amazement of the two brothers. The incident was told with trimmings in the next weekly edition of the Inquirer and Mirror. It is a small world these days!

Before closing the 1941 episode I should say that two years later I operated on Mr. Gade. When I refused to send him a bill because of our mutual friendship and experience in the Mediterranean area, he sent me a beautiful silk Kirman rug, which decorated my study for many years and always reminded me of the interesting interlude during my hectic efforts to get home.

Again, I have gone ahead of my story. In 1936, when we were giving examinations for internships at the Presbyterian, a young man appeared saying that he had been working at the Rockefeller Institute with Carrel [4], and had been advised by him to apply for surgical training under me. He was a Bavarian, and while working in Copenhagen, he had met Carrel and Lindberg [5] and had become interested in the work they were doing with their heart pump. At that time we had an arrangement for some of the appointees to take a year in laboratory work before beginning their surgical training. When Richard Bing [6] had passed the examination, I asked him if he would like to continue his study of the heart pump in the physiology laboratory at P & S for a year. He accepted this appointment and after he had started his work I began to hear interesting things about him; his rare accomplishments as a pianist, as well as his ability as a research worker.

Sis had been working in the hematology laboratory during that year, especially in connection with the patients in the Spleen Clinic and had become very proficient in blood studies that are so important in the diagnosis of spleen disorders. I had given her a fine Leitz microscope, which she used in her work in the laboratory.

One afternoon my secretary said that Dr. Bing wished to see me, so I asked him to come into my office in the Harkness Pavilion where I had been seeing private patients. He came in and said that he had a very special request to make. He said that before proposing to my daughter he very urgently wanted my consent to do so, that he had come to know her as a very lovely young lady, and was convinced that their future happiness would be determined by one thing only. Coming as such a complete surprise, this request left me speechless for a moment, but I said I appreciated his coming to see me first, and that after talking to Sis and mum I would give the matter every consideration.

Mum and I soon found that Sis was as much in love with Richard as he was with her, and that their engagement was the one thing in the world that she wanted. So it was agreed that after a sufficient time for them to be sure of themselves and for us to get better acquainted with Richard, we would, make the announcement and a later marriage date would be set.

We soon realized why Sis was so attracted to Richard, for his visits to our home, his fine musicianship, his great culture and his experience in the European centers, as well as his charming personality convinced mum and I that Sis had made no mistake in her discriminating choice. Although Richard spoke English correctly, he was not too familiar with some of our American idioms. One morning he had breakfast with mum, and us looking at some overdone toast, asked him if he would care to take some of the vile toast. Apparently his thoughts were not on the quality of the article, but later he told us that at a restaurant at breakfast he asked the waitress to bring him "some vile toast" and did not understand her surprised expression when she asked him why he wanted that kind!

Richard became so interested in the research he was doing in the laboratory that he decided to continue in physiology. I agreed with him and urged him to go on with the original work that he was doing. Certainly his remarkable career in the study of the heart, its physiology and disorders, has vindicated him in his decision, for now he is acknowledged as one of the eminent leaders in that field, both in this country and abroad.

Footnotes

1. **Myron Charles Taylor (1874-1959)**
   American industrialist and diplomat who also practiced law and ran textile mills in New England. Between 1939 and 1950 Taylor was the President's personal diplomatic representative to the Vatican, Rome.

2. **Eugenio Pacelli - Pope Pius XII (1876-1958)**
   The Pope during WW II.

3. **John A. Gade (1875-1955)**
   An American banker who was sent to Belgium in 1916 by the "Commission of Relief for Belgium". In 1933 he became the military attaché for the US Navy in Brussels. He published his experience as a navy intelligence officer in his book *All My Born Days*. New York, Scribner, 1942.

4. **Alexis Carrel (1873-1944)**

   A pioneer in vascular surgery. Born in Lyon, France, where he completed his medical education. His interest in anatomy and operative surgery developed in the laboratory of the anatomist Jean-Léo Testut in Lyon, France, where he described his results with suturing of blood vessels. In 1904, after a year of advanced medical studies in Paris, he immigrated to North America and settled in Chicago where he conducted numerous experiments in vascular surgery and transplantation. He continued his work at the Rockefeller Institute in New York and won the Nobel Prize in 1912 for medicine "in recognition of his work on vascular suture and the transplantation of blood-vessels and organs."

5. **Charles Lindberg (1902-1974)**

   An American pilot and inventor best known for his first non-stop flight across the Atlantic Ocean (1927). He, along with Dr. Alexis Carrel, developed the first artificial heart and lung machine. He received a Congressional Medal of Honor and the Distinguished Flying Cross from President Coolidge. Lindberg was a Pulitzer Prize winner (1954) for his autobiography *The Spirit of St. Louis*.

6. **Richard Bing (1909-)**

   See dedication.

Chapter Sixteen

World War II

1939 - 1945

The next summer we spent July and August in the Corscaden cottage in Nantucket, as we had leased ours for the season. Sis and Richard visited us in August, the month that the terrible World War II started, worse than the first. It was a dreadful announcement that came over the radio, especially for Richard who had experienced the ominous doings of the Nazis while he was in Germany. This, of course, meant that we would ultimately get into the war, and, as before, we were not ready for it. We were more than lucky to have Britain doing such a great job in stemming what at first appeared to be a hopeless tide.

The next October, John, our first grandchild arrived, to the joy of his parents and grandparents. Although he began to speak at an earlier age than usual, he could not say Grandma and Grandpa, but used his own version and ever since we have been called Balmy and Gaddie by all our grandchildren.

In June of 1939 Bumps graduated from Princeton. Among his other extracurricular activities, he had been on the editorial board of the Daily Princetonian, then a much larger and busier board than when I had worked on it. He had written his senior thesis on the International Air Conference in Havana. In order to get at the original documents and the locale of the conference, he and I went to Havana during his Christmas holiday where we had an interesting time getting the material for his thesis. I am sure it was more interesting than my own. We got tired of being solicited for lottery tickets and of hearing the constant tango and other dance music.

At the time he was graduating, our Class of 1904 was having our 35th reunion, so that the family was well represented in Princeton that June. After graduating, Bumps began working at the Chance-Voight Airplane Company near Bridgeport to continue his interest in airplane construction and he began to take his first instruction in flying. A good part of the time he continued to commute from Riverdale to Bridgeport in his car, and he piled up a lot of mileage during the next two years. He was a great comfort to mum during the time I was in Italy, but how he stood the long rides beginning at half past five in the morning and getting back at seven at night was a mystery, but he seemed to thrive on it.

In 1941 it became more and more apparent that we would have to enter the war. Bumps chose the Navy and Henry Shriver the Marines. After I had returned from Italy, Bumps was ordered to Pensacola for training. He came to see mum and I at the Webster Hotel where we were staying before moving back to Haven Avenue and told us that he had proposed to Clemente Brown, whom we all called Minuet. He had come to know her while she was at Sarah Lawrence College. We admired her for her charm, her keen mind, and her sense of humor which matched Bumps'. Like so many other young people at that time, they realized what dangers the future held for them, but they took it like the brave sports they were. Bumps left for Pensacola shortly after that and began his rigid training in flying for the Navy. He found a fine lot of men who became his intimate friends; one of them especially, Foster Fargo.

The years 1940 to 1945 were very busy ones. I was appointed to the Medical Committee of the O.S.R.D., a branch of the National Research Council and later I was Chairman of the Committee on Burns and Contaminated Wounds. This meant that I had to be in Washington at least once a week and sometimes more often. The meetings of this Committee were always too full of agenda and one of the most trying duties as Chairman was trying to finish the agenda in time for the members of the Committee to catch the trains and planes that they had to take to the various cities in the country. They were a fine, select group, most of whom I had known in the surgical societies. We usually had a number of visitors from other committees and from the allied medical officers who came to exchange ideas and experiences from their long fights with common enemies. On December 7th, 1942, mum and I had gone to Wilton to spend Sunday with the Shrivers. That afternoon came the word over the radio that the Japs had bombed Pearl Harbor. We knew that meant immediate and active war and it affected us as it did the people all over the country.

In July of 1943 after a long period of meetings in Washington, I went to Wilton, where mum was staying in the big house. I needed exercise and took it in big doses by scything the grass and weeds around the house and barn. One day I had a long distance call from Dr. Newton Richards, the Chairman of the O.S.R.D. He asked me if I would go to Great Britain and North Africa as a consultant for the National Research Council to study the effects of the use of penicillin, the antibiotic that was being used by the British for the first time in the treatment of war wounds and burns. This was, of course, a command, and I told him that I would be ready in a couple of days. I was given a special passport with a number two priority, which was given only to men on secret missions.

This was especially hard for mum, with Bumps on the Essex in the Pacific and with Sis and her responsibilities with Richard in the Chemical Warfare Division of the Army. But the war was in some of its grimmest phases; everyone had to face the situation. I had little time to do more than arrange for the work at the Presbyterian to be taken over by John and Hugh. One of the medical attendings, Kenneth Turner, had just returned from London as the liaison officer for the O.S.R.D. in Washington. I got very valuable advice from him in the way one had to meet the officials and scientists in London and elsewhere, and the few necessary things to take on the trip. I remember he said the most important article of wearing apparel was a trench coat, and I found he was quite right. Of course I had letters of introduction to many of the British medical officers, and credentials that made it possible for me to go places and see people that would be impossible to reach otherwise.

I left New York on an army plane with several officers and three men from Hollywood who were going over to entertain the G.I.S. One of them was Adolph Menjou [1]. We flew to Ireland and had to stay in Limerick for three days where we got a good idea of the whimsical and shiftless ways of many of the Irish. It was in one of the barrooms in Limerick that those of the party who had not flown the ocean before were initiated into the "Short Snorters" by paying a dollar to all the others who had flown the ocean previously. Having done so before, I started a line of bills to which I added many more on later flights during the trip; some of them being paper money of the North African countries. Another evening some of us attended an Irish version of a circus, which consisted of two clowns, a donkey and a drum and fife, much the most primitive and ridiculous performance that I ever saw.

On reaching London I went to the Park Lane Hotel and that evening as I was crossing one of the avenues, not as yet accustomed to left-hand driving, I suddenly found myself on my back having had my feet knocked from under me by a rapidly disappearing girl on her bicycle. A nice bobby helped me pick myself up and said, "It's a hazardous business, crossing the street at this time of night." I got off with nothing worse than a bruised elbow. The next morning I went to the O.S.R.D. offices and was briefed for my duties and the program that had been arranged for me. It was one that required about five weeks in England and Scotland, with visits to hospitals and laboratories, as well as to the offices of some of the Top Brass in the British Army Medical Corps.

One of the first places I went to was Oxford to see two of the physiologists. This was a happy assignment because the Presbyterian Unit was stationed there and I was able to see all my friends and surgical associates that were training there to become one of the general hospitals to go over to France when the great day would come for the invasion. They gave me a room in the camp and I had a delightful time in the canteen, meeting all the doctors and nurses whom I had known so well. One of the most interesting experiences was sitting with them listening to the B.B.C. at six o'clock, to hear the news of the war and the results of the bombing that the British and American flyers were doing everyday in enemy territory. Every evening at dusk we heard and saw from 80 to 120 B29s flying over Oxford on their way to the targets after leaving their airdromes in England.

Of course I had messages from the people at the Presbyterian to members of the Unit, and carried back messages to their dear ones in New York. This was only one of three trips that I made to Oxford, all of them interesting. The food at the Unit canteen was a blessing after the rationed food that I had been getting everywhere in England and Scotland. The only two eggs that I had during my entire stay in Great Britain and Africa were given us at the home of Sir James Learmonth [2], Professor of Surgery at the University of Edinburgh. He had asked me to stay in their home while I was in that city for two days. Mrs. Learmonth was an American whom he had met when he was working at the Mayo Clinic.

One Sunday I had to spend in Bristol and another in Aberdeen; both of these cities were very Presbyterian and nothing in the way of amusement was allowed. In both places it rained so hard that one could not walk in or about the town. In Aberdeen I caught a bad cold, or it caught me, so that I have no pleasant memories of that Granite City.

Sir Henry Dale [3], the President of the British Research Council, invited me to dinner at the famous Atheneum Club, which I found with some difficulty because of the blackout. This was a constant problem at night and made night excursions of any sort very uncertain and unpleasant. Sir Henry advised me to go to North Africa, where they were beginning to use penicillin in war wound treatment. For this trip I had to get permission from the American Army. This was given in a permit signed by General Eisenhower.

Queues and afternoon tea were the most characteristic features of the Londoners. I remember one night during the blackout when I had called on a man in the city. After leaving him, I stood at a bus stop and a man approached and asked, "Are you a queue?" There was a definite understanding that one had to stand in line, and anyone trying to break into it was made to know that it was not cricket, in no uncertain terms, and had to go back to the end of the line. How the taxis managed to travel through the dark of the blackout I could not understand. One of the drivers told me that they found their way around by seeing the silhouettes of the tops of the buildings.

An excerpt from a letter that I wrote to Eunice may be of interest: "The purpose of my mission was to study penicillin, especially the local application of it in the treatment of wounds and burns. Because of the scarcity of penicillin in Great Britain, they had been using it in the treatment of many cases of severe bums in their Air Force; whereas in the States we have had a greater experience in the use of it intravenously for blood stream infections. To get what I needed in methods of its local use, I had to go to a good many hospitals and laboratories, especially the military ones where they had been using it on the burned airmen. There is plenty of red tape connected with such a tour of inspection, and the British are proper sticklers for protocol and credentials; in the war they have to be. This required making appointments, which could not be done in a hurry. They are charming and most courteous and hospitable once you have been given the proper entree. As a result, I met all kinds of brass hats and high officials, making some very happy acquaintances and renewing many old ones.

"One of the most important centers to study of burns is in the Royal Infirmary in Glasgow - the hospital where Lister made his profound studies in antiseptic surgery. Colebrook [4], who is in charge of the Burn Unit there, is a delightful fellow, with whom I had corresponded a great deal as Chairman of the Burn Committee in Washington. So we had a great deal in common and exchanged our ideas and experiences.

"Scotland is just as whimsical and individual as ever. To hear the Scots burring is worth the trouble of getting there. The war has made it hard to get hotel and sleeper accommodations, so I have spent a number of grim nights on lounges and seats on the trains.

"London is in many ways more interesting than ever, but in a tragic way. It shows the effect of the Blitz more than any other city, and it is amazing how the Londoners have accommodated themselves to the damage and the housing shortage. One of the most astonishing sights is to see the many people sleeping in metal triple-deckers in the subway stations. These people have been bombed out of their homes and have found the subways the only available place to sleep and they don't have to worry about the bombs any longer, for the subways are used as shelters.

"The other night some sixty German planes came over the East coast, with fifteen of them flying over London. The hundreds of searchlights and barrage balloons were an astonishing sight. The planes were flying from sixteen to eighteen thousand feet high, but even at that distance, shells from the ack ack guns could be seen exploding around the planes. Three of them were shot down. The others dropped bombs that blew up several houses in one of the suburbs. Unless there are a great many planes overhead, the people don't go to the shelters, and now the Nazis do not have the large number of bombers that they once did. I was in Simpsons the night these planes were over London, having dinner with one of my former residents. When we heard the sirens, the waiter said, 'There go the Jerries again,' and went on with his work as if nothing were happening.

"The rationing of food and everything else in clothing and shoes is very strict. This has made everyone feel that it is done fairly, with no favorites, rich or poor. One cannot get more than a soup, an entree, and either a sweet or a savory (pudding or tart). Tea is rationed, as are sugar and butter. There is very little fruit to be had. A bunch of grapes that I saw on a peddler's cart on Oxford Street was priced at 17/6 - $3.00. Oranges are only for children. The bread is whole wheat, but very edible and uniform. They also handle their labor well. If a man or woman gives up a job, they are apt to find themselves on a farm or at an essential job whether they like it or not."

The African part of my mission, where I went to study fresh war wounds acquired in Sicily and Italy, proved most interesting in many ways. It was totally different from the United States and Great Britain in climate, terrain and population, for in addition to the native Arabs, one saw thousands of soldiers and officers of all the Allies except the Russians. After I had seen my travel permit I went to Prestwick, in Scotland. There was frost on the ground the night we took off for Morocco in an army bucket-seat plane. In the morning we landed in the desert, outside the ancient walled city of Marakesh in summer heat. Of course many of the sights, sounds and smells reminded me of my early Persian days. The morning after we had arrived, I was awakened at dawn by the familiar sound of the muezzin giving the call to prayer from one of the minarets in the town. For a long time, probably not more than a few seconds, I could not imagine where I was.

It was a sight to see - caravans of camels, donkeys and horses on either side of the main highway, with jeeps, tractors, trucks and gun carriages roaring through the middle. While in Marakesh I met an interesting Oxford graduate who was coming up from Khartoum as a casualty on his way to England. We were both in mufti so that we could go into the walled town, which was out of bounds for the military. In one of the main squares of the city they were having a celebration for the end of Ramadan, and annual month of fasting. Here were all kinds of shows, some bad, others much worse, as well as snake charmers. While we were watching the latter, one of the charmers came up to me holding a cobra in his hand and said, "This is a deadly serpent." I asked him where he had learned to speak English; he replied that he had worked at the New York World's Fair. The Englishman told me some very amusing things about Gilbert, of Gilbert and Sullivan, while he was spending the winter in Marakesh. Some of Gilbert's limericks were very funny, but had never been published, for they never would have passed the censor. My most interesting experience was the ten days that I spent with the Second Auxiliary Unit in the Biserte area. The city itself had been frightfully bombed and shelled by several invading forces - Italian, German, British and American. This area was then the center of supplies for Italy, and the American hospital area for receiving the casualties from Sicily and Italy. There were five general hospitals of 1000 beds each, four station hospitals, and two evacuation hospitals, all having some 6000 wounded in various stages of healing and convalescence. It was amazing how quickly these tented units were put up and functioning. One of these from Albany that I saw was set up in the desert area in three days and was caring for 1100 patients. Both doctors and nurses were doing a fine job under the handicaps of sand, mosquitoes and flies.

Fortunately for me the consulting surgeon for North Africa was my friend Edward Churchill [5], who had been a member of the Committee in Washington and the Surgical Chief at the M.G.H. in Boston. He gave me every facility for studying war wounds. I shared his tent and the officers' mess. He took me with him and his two associates (I called them the

"Three Musketeers"), on their rounds of the American hospitals in the Bizerte area, and, later in my stay, I had a chance to see a number of British and French hospitals, but found them inferior to ours. There was little to see in the city itself except ruins and rubble. It was the worst bombed place that I saw during my entire tour.

I had to spend a few days in Algiers, before and after leaving Bizerte, and found that city a bad combination of French and Arab living. The hotel that had been set-aside for American officers was one to forget. When I got a permit to fly back to Scotland, I took another bucket-plane that was carrying a number of wounded soldiers in one kind of splint or another. The poor lads that had airplane splints for fractured arms had the most uncomfortable time of it.

Another week in London, during which time I went to Bocking to try to find if there were any of the Whipple clan living there. I took a train to Prestwick and after waiting there for a couple of days, I took off with a number of officers and war correspondents. We had to land in Iceland because of the weather and spent the night in a Nissen hut, which was chained to the ground with several iron cables to prevent it being blown away by the very strong prevailing winds. The next morning when I was in the men's room shaving I heard a magnificent baritone coming out of one of the showers. Soon a fine looking man came out and said good morning. I returned the greeting and after he had asked my name he said, "I am Masaryk [6], the son of the President of Czechoslovakia. I have escaped from the Nazis with only this," pointing to his somewhat rotund abdomen. Later I found him on the plane to New York, seated next to John Steinbeck [7], the two of them having seen much of each other during the war.

Later in December we had a long distance phone call from Bumps who was in San Francisco. He said that he had been ditched in the Pacific with an injury to his left hand, and had been sent home. But he said he was not badly injured. He arrived in New York two days later to meet Minuet at the Waldorf Astoria where they stayed for a few days. We had Hugh Auchincloss examine Bumps' hand. He operated and found that there was a compound fracture of the index finger of the left hand, with an injury to the flexor tendon. Because of the extensive scar tissue and infection, Hugh was unable to get the finger back to normal and ever since Bumps has had some permanent flexion of the injured finger as a memento of a serious accident that took him out of active fighting on the Essex and sent him homeward to Washington for another two years of duty in the Navy.

The accident was the result of his having to fly on patrol duty in a plane that was not his regular one. He had two other men with him as they cruised fifty miles beyond the Essex, in enemy waters, looking for Japanese planes. Something went wrong with the ignition system, resulting in loss of control of the plane. He, being the pilot, had to pancake into shark-infested water and, because they were in Enemy Ocean, he could not radio to the Essex. The only thing they could do was to blow up their May West jackets, turn on their backs, and wait for their bombs to go off after the plane had sunk a certain distance away. When they did explode, the men were shot out of the Pacific many feet into the air. Bumps wryly said they felt bolter, although badly jarred, because they knew the sharks would be out of business in that area. One of the men could not inflate his jacket; he said that it was the third time for him and that he was out, but the other two would not let him sink and held him up for an hour or more until a motor boat from the Essex was sent out to look for them when the plane had not returned and they were rescued. It must have been a very harrowing experience for Bumps and his crew.

My work in the hospital was very active in revising the residency-training program to accommodate the men who had left the training during the war, and had returned to complete their required duties. There were many fascinating stories that they had to tell about their experiences, all the way from conquered Germany to Guadalcanal and beyond to Iwo Jima to Japan. It was so gratifying to find how well they picked up where they had left off, and with the restricted program that was necessary to give them work as well as to the men who had been appointed during their absence.

We also had to revise the curriculum of the medical school with the members of the other departments back to the four-year program, for

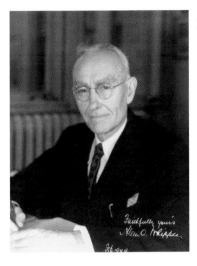

Dr Whipple in 1945.

during the war we had been doing what the other medical schools had done, working on an accelerated schedule of three years. It was such a pleasure and relief to have men like Barclay Parsons, Larry Sloan, Pete Rousselot and Rudy Schullinger [8] back with the staff. They had served with distinction and deserved a special accolade for the work that they had done in and out of the Presbyterian Unit.

It was becoming more and more evident that the time for my retirement, after twenty-five years as Head of the Surgical Department, was approaching, and I began giving the matter of future plans serious thought. I felt that it was important to leave the Presbyterian and Columbia, so that my successor would have a free hand. I had seen the mistake of not doing so in other departments.

Footnotes

1. **Adolph Menjou (1890-1963)**
   Born in Pittsburgh. A movie star also known as one of the best-dressed men in Hollywood. His autobiography *It Took Nine Tailors* was published in 1948.

2.   **Sir James Learmonth (1895-1967)**

Chairman of Surgery at the Royal Infirmary of Edinburgh and the surgeon to King George VI. He reported the first Transverse Carpal Ligament (TCL) release to treat median nerve compression at the wrist.

3.   **Sir Henry Hallett Dale (1875-1968)**

A pharmacologist who received the Nobel Prize in 1936 for his work on the chemical transmission of nerve impulses. He is the author of *Adventures in Physiology* (1953), and *An Autumn of Gleaning* (1954).

4.   **Leonard Colebrook (1883-1967)**

A bacteriologist who was in charge of the Burn Unit at the Glasgow Royal Infirmary. Under him, the unit became a Medical Research Council project. It was during this time that Tom Gibson carried out his work on the "second set phenomenon". Peter Medawar, later Sir Peter, was brought to the Unit to carry out further work with Gibson, which formed the basis of present day tissue transplantation. Medawar was awarded the Nobel Prize (1960).

5.   **Edward D. Churchill (1895-1972)**

A pioneer thoracic surgeon, John Homans Professor of Surgery at the Harvard University Medical School and Chief of the General Surgical Service at Massachusetts General Hospital. He served as a Chief Surgical Consultant to the US Army in the North African-Mediterranean Theatre during WW II. His contribution to military surgery is summarized in his book *Surgeons to Soldiers* (1972).

6.   **Jan Masaryk (1886-1948)**

A diplomat, an ambassador and later on the Czechoslovak foreign minister; the son of Tomas Garrigue Masaryk, the first President of independent Czechoslovakia, that came into existence in 1918. Jan Masaryk was found dead under the bathroom window of his flat; the cause of his death has been shrouded in mystery.

7.   **John Steinbeck (1902-1968)**

An American novelist, storywriter, playwright, and essayist. Steinbeck received the Nobel Prize for literature in 1962. During WW II he served as a journalist - a period covered in his book *Once there was a war* (1958).

8.   **Rudolph N. Schullinger (1896-1969)**

A Professor of Clinical Surgery at the P & S of the Columbia University. As a Colonel in the US Army during WW II, he became the Chief of Surgery at the Presbyterian Hospital Military Unit.

Chapter Seventeen

Retirement and the trip
to the Middle East

1946

In July 1946, when I had reached the retirement age of 65, Dusty Rhoads [1], the Director of the Memorial Hospital and the Sloan-Kettering Institute in New York, visited me. He made me the offer of Clinical Director of the Memorial Hospital. I told him that Mary and I had planned to go to Beirut for several months, where I had promised to act as visiting surgeon in re-organizing the surgical department in the American University, and that if the offer at the Memorial held, I would not be able to give my entire time to the job, as I had certain commitments that would require my giving some time to them. He said that this could be arranged and would be agreeable to them, so I agreed to come to the Memorial Hospital on our return from Beirut.

For several years I had been on the Board of Trustees of the American University of Beirut and was familiar with many of their problems. The Board was sending Mary and I to Beirut, paying our expenses there and back, and had provided a house for us to live in while we were there. I had persuaded Joe MacDonald [2], one of my recently graduated residents, and one of the ablest of the many men who had trained under me, to go to Beirut to take charge of the surgical department for a period of three years. He and his wife, Joe Jeanette, left for Beirut about three months before we left for that city.

The leave-taking at the Presbyterian and the medical school was made easier and also memorable for me by the farewell dinners and the silver pieces that the surgical staff and the faculty gave to me: a large cigarette box from the residents, a beautiful Tiffany gold watch and chain from the attending surgeons, a large bowl from the faculty, and a silver platter from special friends of the medical service, the surgical service and the administration of the hospital.

Mary and I had plenty to do in leaving the house in Riverdale and in packing two trunks for the stay in Beirut. But we were ready by the end of September and had engaged passage to England on the Queen Mary. A strike at the docks in New York made it necessary for us to go to Halifax to get the boat. Jack and Bumps came to the train to see us off for Halifax, which we reached after a stupid, slow train ride of 24 hours.

Sis had saved the letters that we had sent from Beirut, and I am using part of them to tell of our doings after we left the Queen Mary. The trip on the boat was comfortable. We had dinner with the ship's surgeon, and there met the Lord High Chancellor of England. The General Eisenhowers were on board, but kept to themselves on the top deck. After reaching Southampton we took the train to London.

As always, seeing London was thrilling, but the damaged and wrecked houses and stores, where whole blocks were in ruins, was a grim reminder of what I had seen in '43, but new to mum. The outlook for the British must have been dark for both the present and the future. One sees it in the faces of so many, especially the older people. London looks shabby and that hurts the Londoners.

We went to Simpsons for dinner, but found a very different place from that in 1930. The menu had three choices: chicken, tripe, and cold gosling. They had run out of jugged hare, and the chicken resembled an old rooster. The waiters, the white-capped chefs and the silver salvers on wheels were still to be seen, but all had a dejected look. The food in London was worse than when I was there during the war. The bread was rationed and was not so palatable. Butter, meats and sugar were all very limited, but they still had plenty of porridge for breakfast.

The next letter was from the Middlesex Hospital. "The heading of this letter must not alarm you. I am here in mum's private room, where she has been during the last week because of a flare-up of her eczema. The dermatologist we consulted said the condition required hospitalization before we go to the Near East. The strenuous days in London, especially in trying to get some of the necessary clothing as a result of the lost suitcase, has been the cause of the return of the eczemas. She is so much better and has had a good rest with very good nursing. She is all for the English Sisters. But the thing that made it hard was giving up the trip to Paris (more of which later) for she had always loved that city and had looked forward to the festivities and entertainments of L'Academie de Chirurgie to which I had been appointed as the U.S. delegate.

"But first I must tell you about the dinner and ceremony of my induction as an Honorary Fellow of the Royal College of Surgeons of England, which took place on October 1st. I had been in correspondence about this with Sir Alfred Webb-Johnson [3], the President of the College, in the previous spring. He had asked me to accept the Honorary Fellowship the next time I came to London. He said he was anxious to have the induction before a number of their members had to leave for the meetings in Paris, so he called the Fellows in London and, astonishingly enough, arranged the dinner for the next evening. Because of the loss of the suitcase, mum had no evening gown, and when I told Sir Alfred of our catastrophe he said, 'My dear fellow, you know since the war we do not always dress for dinner, so don't give it another thought.' I learned afterwards that he had telephoned every one of the Fellows and their wives to tell them not to dress for dinner to avoid embarrassment to mum. The next evening all the ladies arrived in day dress, the men wore their fellowship gowns, including myself while being inducted.

"Mum had a very nice black afternoon suit, and looked better than any of the other twenty wives. We met first in the secretary's room for sherry, where I was given the red-bordered gown and signed the book. This gave us the opportunity to meet the host and Lady Webb-Johnson and the Fellows and their wives, many of whom I had met either in the States or in England during the war. They were the most distinguished and delightful group of people.

"We then went into the Surgeon's Hall with its magnificent dining table, covered with the ancient and beautiful silver service. Some of the pieces dated back to the time of Henry the Eighth. The walls, recently renovated and re-lighted following the damage done by Nazi bombing of the building, were lined with portraits, which had been stored during the Blitz. These were of famous surgeons, members of the College, painted by Reynolds, Rayborn and Lawrence, a museum of art in themselves.

"Mum and I sat on either side of Sir Alfred, the President, who turned to mum and said, 'How charming you look.' We were never more cordially and royally entertained. Everything was so perfectly done: the service, the conversation, the introduction of the new Honorary Member by Sir Heneage Ogilvie [4], and the induction by Sir Alfred, with the presentation of the inscribed scroll of fellowship to the embarrassed, but greatly appreciative, new member. Mum was her most charming self, and I was never more thrilled and honored. We were quite overcome by the cordiality of their members, as well as by the distinction of the rare occasion.

"Two days later we called on Sir and Lady Gordon-Taylor [5] who had been so kind to me when I was in London during the war. We took her some apple blossom bath salts and powder that I had bought in New York and which Sir Gordon had told me she was so fond of. She appreciated this very much as it was difficult to get such luxuries in England at that time. She was a remarkable woman, an artist and expert on such things as petit point work and Japanese lacquer. During the war they were bombed out of their home on two occasions, and she told the most amazing stories about her work as a first aid worker in the bombed areas; she worked at times three or four days without a chance to rest or change her clothes."

The next letter home was from Cairo and read as follows: "October 23rd, 1946. Our last letter was written shortly after I had returned from Paris, in the evening. I went directly to the Middlesex Hospital to find mum much better and in very good spirits. She was enthusiastic about the treatment they had given her, especially of the nursing. But it was not

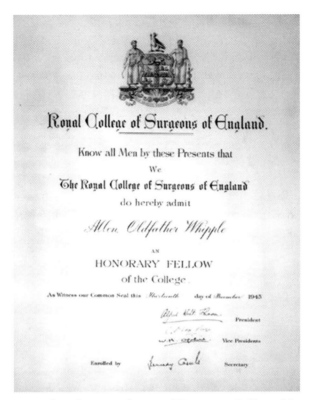

Dr. Whipple's certificate of Honorary Fellowship granted by The Royal College of Surgeons of England.

until two days later that they let her return to the hotel. In the meantime I was able to contact a number of men in cancer work in preparation for my duties at the Memorial Hospital.

"The week in Paris was supposed to be given over to the three sessions of L'Academie de Chirurgie of France in celebration of the centenary of that august institution. But the so-called sessions, supposedly scientific, were made up largely of orations in French and a large part of the time was spent in attending dejeuners and dinners at the homes of the leading French surgeons. At the end of the five days I, as well as the group of British surgeons with whom I stayed at the Hotel Regina, was completely fed up with the black market, French cooking and wining. Champagne twice a day for five days was enough of too much.

"Two or three of the ceremonies were especially formal. The first, a dinner to honor the visiting surgeons given by the French government at the Salon des Allies was official and rather stuffy. Medals were presented to the nine foreign surgeons who were elected members of the Academy. The second was the dinner given by L'Academie at which the newly elected members made speeches in French acknowledging the honor. My friend, M. Bonset who had visited us at the Medical Center last summer, reviewed my speech, made some corrections, so that my British associates were surprised and accused me of having kept my light under a bushel. But it is a bit terrifying to give a speech in a foreign language, in such an assembly. Mine had the virtue of brevity. My previous stays in France and my early lessons in French gave me an advantage in pronunciation over the other British who had never been distinguished for their French. They hemmed and hawed and use their own pronunciation of the French words. The toastmaster was old M. Hartmann [6] who got the names of the speakers well jumbled. He called me Sir Max Page of London, to the annoyance of Sir Max.

"The last ceremony was on Thursday afternoon when L'Academie convened in the great Salle of the Hotel de Ville for their final meeting and the induction of the new foreign members. The Salle was decorated in the Louis Seize period with all the pomp and ceremony that only the French can put on. Long orations by three of the officers of L'Academie, read from printed copies, long and tiresome, were especially annoying to the British. The newly elected members responded to the reading of their names by presenting to L'Academie a scroll, some of them very elaborately engraved on vellum, expressing their appreciation and good wishes to the members of L'Academie. It was a typical formal French performance, without a touch of humor for those who did not take it too seriously. The whole technique and philosophy of the French is so different from that of the British in their induction of new members. The British have great ceremony, as shown at the dinner of the Royal College of Surgeons of England the week before, but it was done so easily and genuinely. With the French there is too much flowery oratory and too little organization.

"Mum came back from the hospital, her eczema almost gone, which she attributes to Johnson's Baby Powder, recommended to her by her favorite nursing sister. Notwithstanding our efforts, we were unable to unite English coupons with London prices to make up for the lost wardrobe in the stolen suitcase. Our coupons for 'sweets' we found had expired before mum left the hospital, and since then we have been unable to get even a lollipop.

"Sunday morning we left London for Cairo by plane via Marseilles, Malta and Libya. Before reaching Marseilles we ran into a thunderstorm; the plane was struck by lightning, which knocked out the compass. After landing on the airfield in Marseilles we were told that the plane would not be able to fly until the next morning, and we were driven to a small hotel outside the city. The next morning, at five, we were driven to the airfield and were off for Malta. We passed over Corsica and Sardinia, which brought back unhappy memories, and by noon we reached Malta. It is a unique little island in the Mediterranean, the most thoroughly bombed area during the war. We were too far out of the town of Malta to see much of the damage. After lunch we were off again, and by four p.m. we were skirting the coast of Libya, passing over the much-contested strip on the parts of the Italian, German and British armies. Finally we passed over El Alamain and the Nile Delta with its myriad lights between Alexandria and Cairo.

"We reached the Cairo airport by about eight o'clock, but were not met by the agent as we had expected. I had started to have a session with the impolite custom officials when a rotund Egyptian introduced himself as Mr. Samara. He said he had been trying to get in touch with me for two days and had learned that I was on my way to Cairo. He had cabled about his son who had an abdominal tumor and wanted me to come to Cairo for a consultation. Meeting me while I was struggling with the custom officials did not make me a very cordial consultant, but when he quickly got our baggage O.K.'d by a mere wave of his hand, and also offered to take us to the Continental Hotel in Cairo, he immediately became our good angel, especially when he gave me a lot of Egyptian currency and placated several porters and bakhsheesh with extended palms. He brought us to the hotel in his Packard car; he said the Continental was less contagious than the famous Shepherds. By a mere gesture he got us a comfortable room with bath, which we could not have had, without his influence.

"Mr. Samara turned out to be a graduate of the American University of Beirut (A.U.B.) in Beirut and a very well-to-do and influential citizen of Cairo. I saw his son in consultation with the Egyptian surgeon who was experienced and competent. He had explored the son and had found a serious and inoperable tumor. I was able to assure Mr. Samara that everything had been done for his son that could be done.

"The Samaras asked us to have lunch in their home the next day, and he arranged to have some of my American Express checks exchanged for Egyptian money at a much better rate than we could have done at the hotel or bank - black market, no doubt. That afternoon we got a car and an excellent dragoman and visited the great mosque with its superb minarets, and then drove across the Nile to the pyramids and the sphinx. One hears so much about these ancient monuments that we were prepared to be disillusioned. But there is no doubt that when one gets close to them and sees the enormous blocks of stone so accurately placed - some 2,500,000 one and one quarter ton blocks are said to have been used in building the Great Pyramid - one begins to appreciate the grandeur and the tragedy of human effort, so long before the machine age, and at the expense of human life. Some 5,500 years old, the Great Pyramid and the Sphinx, sand and weather worn, stand wonderfully impressive.

"If you could have seen mum and I on camels approaching the Sphinx! I hope the Kodak picture I took of mum on her camel turns out well. Certainly, brilliant sunlight was not lacking. The day was a perfect Nile day, the sunset behind the Great Pyramid could not have been more gorgeous as we sat before the cafe and listened to the dragoman's stories. Another blessing was the absence of the Cairo flies, which are the most numerous and sticky that I have ever seen in the East.

"The next day we visited the National Museum and toured the bazaars. Mum seemed to stand the Eastern dirt and smells better than I expected. In fact, I had to urge her to keep going, for she was fascinated by the unusual sights and scenes in the bazaars. In the National Museum they have a unique collection of Egyptian antiquities, including the entire collection of the contents of the tomb of Tutenkhamen, where he was buried some 4,500 years ago. It contains an unbelievably rich and beautiful group of jewelry, wearing apparel and furniture. The luncheon at the Samaras was a typical, long, drawn-out oriental meal, ending with a Baba Rum and fruit. Mum took some grapes among other non-boiled food."

Footnotes

1. **Dusty Rhoads (-)**

    A pioneer cancer chemotherapist and Director of the Sloan-Kettering Hospital, New York. During the Second World War he headed the US Army Chemical Warfare Service in Washington D.C.

2. **Joseph McDonald (1913-)**

    A Professor of Surgery and the Chairman of Surgery at the American University of Beirut during the 1940s. Later the dean of that medical school.

3. **Sir Alfred Webb-Johnson (1880-1958)**

    President of the Royal College of Surgeons of England. In 1943, he conferred Honorary Fellowship of the College upon Winston Churchill.

4.   **Sir William Heneage Ogilvie, (1887-1971)**

A surgeon at Guy's Hospital, London. The author of several surgical treatises, the most notable being *Surgery Orthodox and Heterodox* (Blackwell 1948). His name is associated with the Ogilvie Syndrome - or colonic pseudo-obstruction.

5.   **Sir Gordon Gordon-Taylor (1878-1960)**

A British abdominal surgeon known for his lifetime interest in Australian surgery. Among his publications: *History of the Second World War Surgery* (1954) and *Sir Charles Bell: his life and times* (Livingstone, 1958). The Royal College of Surgeons of Australia established the "Gordon Gordon-Taylor Medal" for best achievers in boards' examination.

6.   **Henri Hartmann (1860-1952)**

A French surgeon. His name is associated with the Hartmann's procedure, which is widely used in the treatment of left colonic emergencies.

Chapter Eighteen

Lebanon and the Holy Land

1946

"Because we could not get a British plane for Palestine and did not feel like risking an Egyptian one, we decided to take an overnight train to Haifa and then drive by car to Beirut. The ancient Wagon-lit (it must have been discarded by the French or Italians), was no better than the railroad bed. The porter was an ignorant Egyptian Arab, than which there is no worse variety. The dust and heat of the Sinai desert was not kept out of the so-called sleeping car. They called for passport inspection and customs much too often and could not read English, much to our annoyance. Before we left Cairo in the evening, mum was beginning to feel uncomfortable and during the night on the train she had a temperature and had to make frequent trips to a most uninviting 'rest room'. She felt very flat by morning, but the fresh air in the automobile and the drive through Tyre and Sidon along the Mediterranean coast was a welcome change from the dusty train.

"Beirut, October 25th, journey's end. When we reached Beirut we called on President Dodge [1] and his charming wife in Marquand House and were given the warmest of welcomes. Mary Dodge put mum to bed and said, 'You have Gypie Tummy. Everyone coming from Cairo had it.' The doctor in tropical medicine came to see her, put her on a rigid diet and took a culture. It seems everyone coming from Egypt develops a type of bacillary dysentery and, if taken in hand early, recovers rapidly. Having lived in the Middle East in very much the same environment, I must have developed immunity, for I never had any symptoms of the trouble. The next morning mum agreed to go to the hospital, and made a quick recovery.

"The next few days we went to see the Crawfords, whose house we are taking when they go to Damascus. The house is just off the main campus, next to the Boys' School, near the tip of the peninsula. It is a good-sized house with large rooms and high ceilings, and has a beautiful view of the sea and the mountains. Mum is keen about it, and would like nothing better than to refurnish and re-decorate it. The Crawfords, although the finest people and the salt of the earth, do not have mum's taste and distinction. However, it is most comfortable and will soon show mum's touch. The maid and cook, Amenie, is a Druse, one of the Moslem sects, very reliable and speaks English, which is a blessing for mum, as she has no knowledge of Arabic and thinks the language is a most peculiar mixture of gutteral and nasal sounds. Amenie will do the cooking and buying, and her mother will do the housework and washing. She looks like the Witch of Endor, but is a kindly soul. Beirut is largely a Moslem community, and one hears evidence of it five times a day. There is a minaret over a mosque about a block from our house from which the call to prayer is given five times a day. The muezzin, the man giving the call, has a fine, melodious voice and gives the 'azan' well, but mum can't pronounce the name and calls him the Moo.

"Yesterday I made rounds with Joe MacDonald. He has already more than made good and has already established a reputation. There are more than one of the Presbyterian nurses here, and the anesthetist, Miss Meyers, worked with me at the Medical Center. There will be much making and returning of calls, which will establish the afternoon habit with us. We have already had dinner and reception invitations and there will be few dull moments. But we miss letters from home; this is a far place from home and the family and we have many moments of nostalgia.

"Sunday, November 10th. It is now more than two weeks since we arrived and we are now well settled in the new home, with the trunks here. Our engagement calendar is fairly full, for the people, native and American, are very cordial. The Dodges gave a big reception for us to which some 200 of the A.U.B. professors and associates came - a most interesting, but confusing group of names and faces, and a good cross-section of the people working in the university. This is a university in every sense of the word; some eighteen nationalities are represented.

Teachers and students have come here from all over the Near and Middle East as well as from Greece, Turkey, Egypt and Ethiopia, for a definite purpose. Along with the teaching and learning, there is some research going on, with the need for much more.

"The campus here is one of the most striking and beautiful in the world, with such magnificent views of sea and mountains. Certainly no more unusual flora can be seen on any campus, such as trees like the banyan from India, eucalyptus from Australia, mimosa from the Pacific, lemon, grapefruit and orange, and the banana from Spain, cedars and pines peculiar to Lebanon, jasmine and chrysanthemums all over the place, and fuchsias and gardenias growing in hedges.

"The lights and shades on the mountain east of us are unique and vary from hour to hour, and from minute to minute at sunset. They are the despair of the amateur landscape painter, and yet a constant invitation. In many ways one is surprised at what he sees on the campus. I have seen as good tennis here as can be seen in international matches. This afternoon mum and I attended a concert of quartet music, a Mozart quartet and a Dvorak quintet done amazingly well by the professional quartet of Beirut. But to go to the concert we had to pass through a primitive part of the town with plenty of dirt, smells and dreariness.

"This morning we went to the Episcopal Church for the commemoration service for the British War Dead. The church is small, but very dignified and the service was most appropriate and well done. In the afternoon we went with the Dodges to the British Veterans cemetery. Nothing could have been more beautiful in scene and service. The British know how to do such things with a sincerity and dignity that is unequalled anywhere else.

"Consultation work has been enough to keep me busy, but a good deal of it is in fields that I am not too familiar with, especially in urology. There is a great deal of kidney and bladder stone disease here, as is the case all through the Near and Middle East. Then I have been asked to give a number of lectures of one kind or another. But I have time to read and paint and we look forward to visiting places like Baalbek and Palmyra before the rainy season begins next month.

"One hears the Lebanese Arabic spoken here by the natives, but it is not the classical Arabic that I studied in Princeton, and which I am starting to take up again with Dr. Nebi Farris. I knew him in the Department of Oriental Languages in Princeton. He is here as a research fellow. His wife is a charming American girl whom he met while in the States. They are living near the mosque, from which the muezzin gives the call to prayer. We are frequently wakened at dawn by his melodious voice which ends the morning call by saying, 'Assalat kheyr min alnum - It is better to pray than to sleep.'

"A member of the staff of the U.S. Ministry and his wife, who is an artist, live in an apartment directly opposite the mosque. They invited us to use their balcony to paint the minaret and the muezzin at the top of it when he was giving the call, so we went there yesterday and I got a good start on a canvas.

"November 17th, 1946. This has been a trying week, for I had to make the decision to operate on Mary Dodge, the President's wife, and the patron saint of this community. She had been losing weight and feeling below par during the summer and her physician feared that she might have a serious abdominal condition. Her x-rays were not revealing, and she had planned to come to New York to see me, but decided to wait until I had arrived.

"Yesterday morning I operated upon her with a full Presbyterian team, Joe MacDonald as my first assistant, Miss Higgins, who had worked with me as an instrument nurse, and Miss Meyers as anesthetist. To my great relief, as well as that of everyone else, we found nothing serious. The loss of their younger son as an airman over Germany during the last war had been a great sorrow to the father and mother, and one that she tried to relieve by ceaseless work, until she had developed an exhaustion state. This operation and the days of her later care and convalescence had prevented our going to Damascus as we had planned, but we hope to make the trip next week, while the wonderful November weather holds out. I have not worn a hat since coming here and am still wearing summer suits.

"Our breakfasts of orange and grapefruit juice from the trees in the yard are always delightful. The chrysanthemums are in their glory and we have hedges of calla lilies blooming. How interested you would be, Jack, in the different varieties of trees and flowers here, for so many of them are very different from those in Connecticut.

"The lack of news from home and the family is the one great trial of being so far away. Not only have we no family news, but also I don't even know who won the baseball championship, to say nothing about the Princeton football scores. The news as it appears on the two page, one sheet daily in English, reports the U.N.O. doings, but mostly with the Arab-Palestine controversy and Soviet propaganda. Except for the A.U.B. and the American work of the University, past and present, the prestige of the United States has suffered greatly, especially with Truman's mistakes and the Democratic defeat, for it is interpreted here as a state of confusion in Washington and the country.

"Beirut, December 1st, 1946. A week ago we went with the Lanes in their car to the lovely bay of Junni, some twenty miles north of Beirut on the Mediterranean coast. While she and I were painting madly, mum read and took in the ablutions of Maronite babies in the Grotto of St. George, just below where we were painting. Mr. Lane made a bluff at a watercolor, but was not so serious as Mrs. Lane and I. We both did a canvas of the bay and the steep Lebanon mountains above it in entirely different styles and got a great kick out of it. Mum is very kind about mine and likes it. The best thing about it is that I finished a fairly large canvas in one sitting, and in a different style from anything that I had done before.

"Friday morning mum and I started on the first real trip out of Beirut in the Dodge's car with their driver who speaks nothing but Arabic. Mary Dodge has done well, but is still convalescing in the hospital, so they are not in need of their car. We went east over the mountain pass down into the Baaka valley, and turned north, on the road to Aleppo. The first stop after a two-hour drive was at Baalbek. This is, in many ways, the most startlingly beautiful ruin of the Greco-Roman temples to be found anywhere. For centuries before the temples were built it had been the site of Phoenician temples to Baal, and was occupied by the Assyrians and Greeks later. Such saints as Commodus built the Roman temples to Jupiter and Baachus! The Mongols, Arabs and earthquakes have destroyed a large part of these temples, but to come off the desert onto these ruins suddenly, with their wonderful remaining facades and pillars, is an experience never to be forgotten. We could not stay more than an hour because of the long trip to Aleppo, but long enough to determine to return for a day later with the MacDonalds.

"The Baaka valley between the Lebanon and the Ante-Lebanon mountains is entirely different from the Mediterranean coast in climate, temperature, terrain and scenery. Much cooler with crisp air, the terrain is desert with oases wherever there is water. The native villages have varying styles: some of them with flat roofs; some, adobe built, are like those seen in New Mexico and others, entirely different, have chocolate-drop like domes, exactly like a collection of bee hives, some of them with doors and some of them with windows. There are no trees, lots of children, sheep, goats, chickens and donkeys wandering about the indefinite streets and alleys between groups of such houses. We were always passing Arabs on donkeys or camels, or flocks of sheep and goats that paid little attention to the honking of the motor horn. Almost always an Arab on the rear end of a donkey leads a string of camels. The reason given for this custom is that the haughty and disdainful camel needs to learn humility by following the lowly ass.

"On the desert we saw a number of Bedouins in one or more black goat hair tents, along with their flocks and camels. These tents are low and seem to be uncomfortable, even more so than the bee hive houses. The Arabs in the villages were plowing their fields with the same primitive ploughs that were used in Biblical times, with a donkey and an ox yoked to the plough. The soil must be rich, for they don't do more than scratch the surface of the fields. We passed through two interesting towns, called Humms and Hammah, both very old and unchanged. The latter is situated on the Orontes River, and has a remarkable pair of huge water wheels that raise the water from the river to the land some eighty feet above. These wheels must be very old, for they look it and make a constant doleful creaking noise.

"By four o'clock we reached Aleppo. This is one of the oldest towns in Syria, and has one of the best-preserved citadels as well as the most interesting bazaars, or 'sooks' as they are called in Arabic. The citadel, or fortress, dates back 4,000 years, first built by the Phoenicians, added to or destroyed by the Egyptians, Assyrians, Greeks, Saracens, Crusaders and by the Mongol Tamurlane. It has now been partially restored to the way it was during the time of the Saracens, and is a most interesting example of the kind of fortress that was used to defend them against the Crusaders. It had a deep moat, crossed by a long bridge leading to the caravan road below. We reached the Hotel Baron at sunset and were surprised to find such a well-run, clean hotel. The owner, an Armenian, had a passion for Persian rugs, and had used them on the floors and walls of the reception room, dining room, and guest rooms and hallways. We were also surprised at the good food they gave us. The next morning one of the Armenians of the hotel guided us through the great citadel and the extensive bazaars. The trip through the miles of these covered bazaars was a weird experience for mum, and for me, a reminder of the same type of structure that I used to see so often as a boy in Tabriz. Mum complained that we were not staying long enough in some of the many sections, such as the silk, leather, wood work, metal work and jewelry. But the walk ways were so narrow and dirty, and the flies so numerous, almost as bad as in Cairo, that I did not think it was safe to spend too much time there. We saw some beautiful silk tent tiles and purchased some brocades for the ladies of the family. But we saw no oriental rugs worth looking at. The next evening we called on Dr. Altounyan [2], an Armenian surgeon, 97 years old, who was the oldest living graduate of the College of P & S in New York; a most remarkably preserved and interesting man. He had established his own hospital and his son was active in it, although the old man was also active in it until he retired at the age of 85.

"On our return from Aleppo, we stopped on the main road to see the famous restored Crusaders' castle, the Krak de Chevaliers. The French did a fine job of restoring this monument of the Crusades. It had been built on the top of a hill that overlooks the entire area for miles around, a very strategic site for the Crusaders who had invaded the Mediterranean coast on their way to Palestine. Surrounded by a deep moat, there are three immense walls encircling the main fort itself, with approaches to the gates in the walls that could be raised in case of attack. The fort itself is an amazing place, with high halls and a deep cistern that collected the water from the deep wells and the rainfall. The fort was made to accommodate more than 5,000 soldiers, and when occupied by the Crusaders, it had enough supplies to last a one-year siege. The famous Kurdish leader of the Moslem forces, Saladin the Great, in the early 1200s A.D, finally captured it.

"This is a challenge for anyone with a paint box and a canvas. I did not have anything more than a piece of plywood board, and the large collection of Arab youngsters that kept surrounding and edging in on the easel, got to be too much of a handicap. So I had to rely on some good photographs that I took for a later attempt at painting the Krak.

"We then returned to Beirut by way of Tripoli and Biblos on the Mediterranean coast. The old ruins of Biblos are the sites of the oldest Phoenician and Hittite civilizations where some of the former Phoenician kings were buried in immense stone sarcophigi. The trip back, except for seeing the Krak, was not as interesting as the one we took to Aleppo, probably because we were surfeited with so many new sights. Then it was the beginning of the rainy season.

"December 10th, 1946. Last week brought us such good letters from home. We felt made over and happy in getting so much home news. During the week we attended receptions given by the alumni of the medical school and the Undergraduate Club of the medical school. Both proved to be interesting affairs, but with so many Arabic names. Because of the last war, postgraduate instruction in the way of clinics and symposia had been discontinued. We were able to announce a new program for giving the newest advances in medicine and surgery. So many of the doctors in this area had not heard of them, or knew very little about such things as chemotherapy, intestinal intubation, early ambulation, the use of silk and cotton in the repair of wounds, and the newer preparations of the anti-malarial drugs. These meetings are to begin this week, with a surgical symposium of three days duration in January.

"At the end of the week Mary and I went to Damascus in the Dodge's car and spent the weekend at the Crawfords, who are living in Damascus this year. They have been coming to our house in Beirut every other weekend, and we have grown very fond of them. They are kindness itself and showed us all around Damascus. The great Umayid Mosque is one of the finest in the Moslem world. It was built in 720 A.D. and was originally a Christian church. Some of the Byzantine Christian mosaics are still to be seen on the walls of the great square of the mosque and over one of the old entrances there is still an inscription which reads, 'Thy kingdom is an everlasting kingdom, oh Lord, and Thy truth endureth from generation to generation.' But the bazaar adjoining it is so built that it can only be seen at certain angles.

"The interior of the mosque is a vast assembly room, with the floor covered with hundreds of oriental rugs; good, bad, and indifferent, which have been donated by the worshippers. At the four corners of the great court are minarets; one of them is called the minaret of Jesus. Of course we had to wear sandals over our shoes before we could go into the court and mosque, most of them were ancient and decrepit.

"The sooks, or bazaars, are not so primitive as those in Aleppo and are not so dirty and smelly because they are not completely roofed over. We saw them blowing glass, making metal trays and bowls, turning wooden articles on their primitive lathes, and using their bare feet and toes as cleverly as their hands. One of the very interesting things to watch was their making and baking the blotting-paper thin bread, as I used to see it done in Persia. Mary was very much taken with their dyeing of yarn and cloth as well as with their weaving. Of course there was the same constant traffic of camels, horses and donkeys and vehicles, ancient and modern, passing through the bazaars, with the honking of horns that must have belonged to Paris taxicabs years ago. The street called 'Straight' that we read about in the New Testament is in a part of the old bazaar, and they point out the window from which St. Paul was lowered in a basket when he escaped from Damascus.

"The city of Damascus, because of the two rivers that flow through it, has a fine water supply, and for over 4,000 years, has been noted for its fine gardens and trees. There is a legend that the prophet Mohammed intended to visit Damascus, but when he saw the city from one of the hills overlooking it, he refused to enter the city; he said he could enter Paradise but once. There are over 300 minarets connected with as many mosques, so that the call to prayer five times a day can be imagined, if not heard. Damascus, said to be the oldest inhabited city in the world, is in many ways the most interesting city in the world, more so than Cairo, Aleppo, and Beirut in the Near East.

"The Dodges plan to be in Luxor, Egypt, during the Christmas holidays, and have offered us their car and chauffeur. So we plan to spend Christmas in Jerusalem and Palestine. They say that there will be no activity of the Stern Gang during the Holy Week, and that travel will be safe during that time. Of course we wanted to have good pictures of this trip. I should have said before this that when I was in Paris and London I had priced Leika cameras, and they asked as much as $200 for a second-hand one. Before we left London I went to the Eastman Kodak people and got a Brownie Kodak for $5.60. It has proven to be so useful, for it needs no light filter or other gadgets, and the enlargements are remarkably good. It had been the best bargain of our trip.

"December 27th, 1946. This letter was written after our return from Palestine. We sent our Christmas greetings to the family from Jerusalem by cable. They were sent under unusual circumstances, which will be mentioned later. The account of the trip must begin with an important circumstance connected with it. Some three weeks ago I had operated on the son of one of the prominent graduates of the A.U.B., Mr. Salami, the representative of the firm of Thos. Cook and Sons, in the Near East. He was an old and experienced guide and was familiar with all the ins and outs of that part of the world. The son had seen a great many doctors, too many, and had planned to come to the States, but waited when he heard I was coming to Beirut. I resected his stomach for a duodenal ulcer and had him out of bed the next day, an unheard of thing in Beirut. He did well, and his father and the rest of the family were amazed and spread exaggerated ideas about the operation and the operator. When the father heard that we were going to Palestine, he insisted on coming with us and giving us the best guided tour as an expression of his appreciation of what I had done for his son. He is a Christian Arab of the Greek Orthodox Church, and his home is in Jerusalem.

"We started from Beirut on the 22nd and traveled by way of Sidon and Tyre, then over the hills of Judea, reaching Jerusalem that evening at teatime. On our way we stopped at Haifa for lunch, where we met Mr. Salami's daughter and son-in-law. We visited the monastery of Mt. Carmel where the prophet Elijah carried out his activities against the Philistine worshippers of Baal.

"The entry into Jerusalem was a sunset, very lovely and impressive. The Salami house was most comfortable and modern, and the servants were most attentive and appreciative of what they thought I had done for the favorite son, George. There was a plethora of oriental rugs, some very good, but draped over chairs and couches, which grieved Mary's sense of color and decoration. The next morning we started to tour Jerusalem with Ibrahim, one of Cook's best Arab guides, first to the Tower of King David, then through the old narrow market of King David Street to the Church of the Holy Sepulcher, where the tomb of Christ is marked by five chapels - Roman Catholic, Greek Orthodox, Armenian, Syrian and Coptic. We then went along the north wall of the city (the walls of Jerusalem are remarkably well preserved, built in 1560 A.D. by Sulaiman the Magnificent) to the Valley of Kedron and up to the Mount of Olives and the Garden of Gethsemane. The Garden is a lovely, quiet spot, cared for by Franciscan monks and is one of unquestioned historic authenticity. Some of the olive trees in the Garden are over a thousand years old, and there are growths of trees that were there at the time of the crucifixion. I had a sketchbook with me and made a drawing of what is said to be the oldest tree. The trunk was well over fifteen feet in circumference, and the tree is mostly trunk, although some of the branches had green leaves on them.

"The Church of Nations just east of the trees is supposed to stand over the rock where Christ prayed apart, while the disciples slept. It is also called the Church of the Agony, and was built in the latter part of the last century from subscriptions from all the Christian nations. For this reason it is unique and without the contentions one sees in so many of the Holy Places.

"Through Bethany and the Wilderness of Judea - and barren and desolate it is - to the Dead Sea, some 1,900 feet below sea level. The water in it is so filled with salt and minerals that it is sticky and has nothing living in it. There are a number of factories on the shore, where they are recovering the salt, phosphate and nitrates for commercial fertilizers and which had been used during the war for munitions. The flat stones on the shore made fine skimmers.

"From there we went to Jericho and the River Jordan. Here they grow a delicious variety of oranges, most refreshing after the hot ride from the Dead Sea. Jericho is entirely an Arab town and has not changed much from the time of Joshua. The Jordan was disappointing for it did not appear to be more than a narrow, muddy stream. The Trans-Jordan Arab guards at the frontier bridge were a crusty lot and forbade our taking any pictures of the Jordan, for no reason that we could learn.

"We returned for lunch at the Salamis where we met a Mr. Blatchford, the uncle of Mary Dodge and Consul General of the U.S. in Jerusalem. He is 78 years old, but active and humorous and whimsical. His knowledge of the city and the people is profound. He seemed to know all the prelates of all the sects, as well as the prominent Jews and Arabs, and had jokes on all of them. His limericks were as funny as they were numerous, some of them a bit risqué, but very apt. He took us with Mr. Salami (they were old friends), to the town of Bethlehem and gave us the entree to many places and people that we would not have seen otherwise.

"The Church of the Nativity, like that of the Holy Sepulcher, is the site of several chapels of various Christian sects. There is much that is tawdry and encrusted with the gifts of the ages. But notwithstanding this, there is a real spirit of holiness and reverence about the site of the manger, as well as the town, that was the beginning of Christianity. The reading of the Nativity in the Gospels, after visiting and seeing Bethlehem, brings out the simple beauty of the story and is refreshing after seeing the embellishments of the centuries in the Church of the Nativity.

"Mr. Blatchford took us to call on the Armenian Patriarch, His Beatitude Brother Cyril, a very impressive long-bearded, and cowled elder, but with a delightful sense of humor, amply stimulated by the stories and quips of Mr. Blatchford, who is his life-long friend. Turkish coffee was served as it is on all occasions here in the Near East. The fact that I had been in Armenia and Persia provided a mutual bond, for the Patriarch was born in Isphahan. From there we went to Mr. Blatchford's home, and then to the Christmas Eve carol service in the Y.M.C.A building. It was in English and was our first real touch of 'home Christmas'. Mr. Salami escorted us to his home, and a real escorting it was, for his house is built across the street from the King David Hotel which had been badly damaged by the Terrorists last summer. British Government officials now occupy the rest of the hotel and the whole area around it, including the Salami house, is surrounded by barbed wire with British troops at regular intervals behind Bren guns. We had passes, but had to show our passports whenever we left or entered the wired area. This evidence of preparedness against the Jewish Terrorists' activities is seen in so many parts of the city, and in other cities in Palestine as well, wherever there are official buildings like railroad stations or post offices. When I took the cablegram, which we sent you for Christmas, to the post office, which was also wired, I had to stop at the entrance, hold my hands over my head and be frisked by a Tommy for a gun or bomb, but this was done with courtesy and efficiency. Everyone, regardless, is treated the same way on entering the building. This makes the visit to Palestine rather grim and makes one realize the seriousness of the situation between the British and the radical Jews. The British are facing the trying task of preserving order between the Jews and the Arabs and getting nothing but hatred from both sides. The United Nations Assembly does not seem to relish the idea of trying to deal with this situation that is full of dynamite and which requires the wisdom of a good many Solomons.

"Both the British and the Americans are very unpopular in the Near East for different reasons. At a dinner that I attended I sat next to a very intelligent Arab. He said he could not understand why Truman and Dewey had behaved as they had in supporting the Jews in their demand to have Palestine, which had been the home of the Arabs for so many centuries. I told him he must realize that this was an election year, and that New York State has a very largely deciding vote, with the Jews controlling it. He must have known that he had me on the hip, and I was stupid to have made this remark, for he said, 'Doctor, you don't mean to say that the candidates for the Presidency would stoop so low as that!' What could I say in reply?

"On Christmas Eve Mr. Salami had some eight people in for dinner, a very cosmopolitan group. A Dr. Cannan, a Christian Arab, was there with his wife, who is a German. They had both been in an internment camp, she for over four years, and he had been in a Turkish prison during the First World War and condemned to be shot. Why he was saved, he never knew. Among his interesting hobbies he had the largest collection of amulets in the world, which he had been collecting for the past thirty years. This he showed us when we called on them the next day and gave us a very interesting talk on the subject.

"We were advised not to try to go to Bethlehem on Christmas Eve because of the uncertainty of the political situation and the great press of the traffic that would be going and coming. So we listened to the carol singing in the Shepherd Field and at the Church of the Nativity that came over the radio. The next morning we looked out of our window and saw the British Tommies across the way from us and gave then a Merry Christmas, which they returned very cordially. They must have been glad to hear a Merry Christmas so unexpectedly.

"The day before Christmas we spent the morning in seeing the Temple area, the name given to that of the Moslem mosques and the site of the rock on which Abraham had started to sacrifice Isaac, although the Moslems say it was Ishmael. It was on this site that Solomon had built the great temple, which had also been restored by Herod. The Omar mosque, or the Dome of the Rock as it is called, is next to Mecca and

Medina, and is considered the most holy place in the Moslem world. It is by far the most magnificent architecturally of any mosque that we have seen, with wonderful mosaics in deep blue and greens. The dome is considered one of the finest in the world.

"On the south side of the temple, the area leads into the Via Dolorama and is near Pilate's house, where Christ was brought to trial and began His walk to Golgotha bearing His cross. The house is now cared for by the Sisters of Zion, a Catholic order. The old excavated Via Dolorosa, a Roman road, is now some 30 feet below the street level and appears to be genuine in every way. The little French nun was a real saint, and impelled all of us, including Simon, the Dodge driver, to feel that we were walking on holy ground. As we walked along this old Via Dolorosa, we suddenly saw a very startling mural, which showed Christ borne down by the cross. Here the Sister paused and asked us to kneel as she offered a prayer in Latin. This was by far the most inspiring place that we saw in all of Jerusalem.

"On Christmas Day we attended the early service at the Anglican Cathedral of St. George. Cannon Bridgeman, brother-in-law of Father Berry in Riverdale, used to be the rector when he lived in Jerusalem. It is a beautiful building, and the service was very appropriate. At noon, after an early lunch, we left the Salamis and started our journey to the Sea of Galilee. At Nablus, after an hour's ride, we came to Jacob's well, where Christ asked the woman of Samaria for a drink of water. This is one of the most authentic of the old places, for it is a very deep well that had been known for centuries before the Christian era, and is known as the well that Jacob gave to his son, Joseph. The water is cold and of fine quality. There is a shrine built over it with the remains of an old Roman church above it. We read the story of the woman of Samaria and Christ and it made our experience very real.

"From there we went to Nazareth and were shown the house of Mary and Joseph and his workshop. Both of these lacked authenticity. It was getting dark so we did not spend much time in Cana, the place where, at the wedding, Jesus turned the water into wine. When we reached Tiberius on the shore of the Sea of Galilee, we were not able to get a room in the main hotel and we had to take one at a very new hotel right on the shore of the lake, or sea. This was an orthodox Jewish establishment and we found that we were the only Gentiles in the place. There were signs posted on the various rooms and the lounge saying that it was the eve of the Sabbath (Friday night) and that smoking was not permitted. The next morning was bright and sunny as we looked out of our balcony opening off our room. From there we saw the old wall of Tiberius, built by the Crusaders, with a round tower near the seashore. Between it and the hotel there was a long Bedouin black, goat-hair tent, with Arab women and children washing and working on the shore. I had my paint box with me and sat on the porch, free from beggars and flies, and settled down to a morning of painting. The piece of plywood, which I had to use in place of a canvas, turned out not too badly; it is still hanging on the wall of my study. It is a reminder of a unique and amusing scene. Here Mary and I saw, between two groups of incompatible Semites, the Arabs and the Jewish crowd in the hotel, a linguistic battle royal. Two Arab harridans and a young crowd of 'city toughs' were shouting at each other. We did not know what the dispute was about, but the Bedouin harridans were holding very successfully and vociferously against more than a dozen of town Arabs. The two Bedouin women were telling them off in vilifying tones, finally driving the townsmen off. I laughed, as did Mary, until my sides ached, for we had never seen more effective viragos.

"That afternoon we had lunch in the home of Mr. Salami's daughter, whom we had previously met in Haifa. Her husband, a physician, drove us to Capernaum and from there, to an old Byzantine church where the mosaic floor had been excavated. This was supposed to be the site of the feeding of the multitude, commemorated in mosaic by the five loaves of bread and two fishes. This was near a new church built by the Italians, on the hillside that is said to be the site of the Sermon on the Mount, and for this reason it is called the Church of the Beatitudes.

"The next afternoon we returned to Cana and were shown the site of the house where the first miracle was performed. The Italian monk took us to a small refectory and gave each of us a glass of Cana wine, which seemed appropriate to the place, although the monk made a claim that the wine had been water - it was rather weak! Cana is a small village with streets barely wide enough for the cars to pass through. The next morning we left for Sidon and Beirut, driving south of snow-clad Mt. Hermon, and through some interesting country. A number of springs emptied into a swampy valley, which was emphatically marked with signs reading 'malarial'. Here we saw many water buffalo plowing the fields, and Arabs weaving mats from the rushes grown in the swamps. This was one of the principal highways between the Mediterranean and Palestine in the days of the contests between the Crusaders and the Saracens. There are several ruins of the Crusaders' castles and forts to be seen along this highway.

"We reached Beirut about noon and were overjoyed to get the letters and cables from the dear ones at home. This was a lonely Christmas for us, but one made memorable by our visit to the Holy Land, and one made so comfortable for us by the use of the car that the Dodges gave us with Simon, the chauffeur. He sang our praises wherever we went. On one occasion when the Cook's representative was guiding us through Jerusalem, the guide turned to us and said: 'Simon tells wonderful things about you. He says you take out peoples' stomach one day and make them walk the day after. No one dies and God is always with you!'

"February 7th, 1947. This is probably the last letter to the family from Beirut, as we hope to be home before another letter can reach you. We plan to leave on the 18th of the month for Cairo, where we have booked flights on a T.W.A. plane to fly via Tunis, Algiers, Lisbon, Shannon and Ganders, to New York. We are packing one trunk and a box containing dutiable things to leave the first of the week; the second one will go after we leave for Cairo.

"I had to go to Damascus for two days in consultation on the President of Syria [3], who has been suffering with a bleeding duodenal ulcer for years, and is obviously in need of surgery. The fact that he cannot drop his work for another month and that I have to leave in two weeks lets me out of a none too welcome operation, for he is not a good risk and would be a problem so far as publicity is concerned. So I advised him to take three months off, come to Washington, ostensibly to call on Truman, and then have the operation in New York, Baltimore, or Boston, as he chose.

My luck in my surgery here has been remarkable, but I feel that I have about used it up. From now on I am turning my patients over to Joe, who also has had equally good luck and has not lost a major case.

"The same evening that I examined the Syrian President, he gave a dinner in honor of George Wadsworth, recently the ambassador to Lebanon, and now on his way to Baghdad in the same capacity. The Prime Minister and other ministers, as well as Bayard Dodge, Archie Crawford, members of the legation, and I were there. The dinner was a very formal affair; white tie and tails, with French food and French was spoken. This was so even though the Syrians hated the French government because of the DeGaulle bombardment of Damascus and the French regime in the French mandate of the past ten years.

"The morning after the dinner I went to the sooks with Mary Crawford and Margie Garrett, the Dodge's daughter. Her husband, John Garrett, is the Pan-American representative in Syria, but he was away in Ankara. We went to parts of the bazaar that I had not seen previously, and came back with a fair amount of loot, some of which I was able to get at very reasonable prices after a good deal of oriental haggling. Margie speaks Arabic like a native, which made the bargaining so much easier.

"The ride back over the mountains was especially beautiful, with bright sunshine overlooking the blue Mediterranean. At the top of the pass we could see many skiers on the miles of snow-covered slopes of varying grades. Some of the skiers had been swimming in the Mediterranean in the morning. As a winter sport, skiing is becoming a favorite, with people coming from Turkey, Egypt and other Arabic speaking countries. I wish I had had more time and more canvasses, for the landscape is so varied and so different from anything we see in the States, but I had done more than a dozen, large and small, in this area. There are so many other enchanting places in the mountains and villages, that one could spend years in trying to capture the mood of this country.

"We find the time too short to do the things we have to do, and yet too long before starting for home. It will be much colder when we return compared to this hybrid country where roses, calla lilies, black iris,

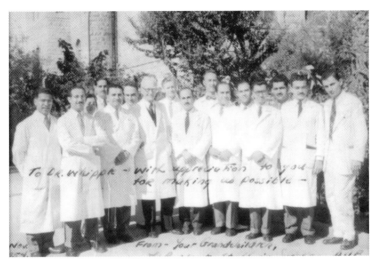

The surgical staff of AUB with Dr. Whipple.

narcissus and nasturtiums are in blossom in our yard. They are the real spring in March, with the wild flowers on the mountains. Altogether, this has been an unforgettable interlude in our lives."

This was the last of the letters from Beirut. Before we left I had written a report for the Board of Trustees, telling of my experience and impressions of the A.U.B. In it I emphasized my appreciation of the past accomplishments of the university and of the great influence that it has had in the past, all through the Near and Middle East. But I also called attention to the fact that times have changed, that the people of these areas were far more intelligent than they had been in the past, and that they expected the university to be as up-to-date as those in Europe and America. There were two things that I emphasized. The first was the need for a greater research program, especially in the area of tropical medicine and in the area of Arab culture. The second was the need for a new library and a change in teaching methods, which were still in the old lecture system. I also called attention to the need for residency training in medicine, which we had started in surgery during my stay in Beirut.

This, in the past, had been entirely neglected. The last matter to which I called attention was the vicious habit of shopping on the part of patients in the Near East; the patients went from one physician to another, with useless and confusing duplication of laboratory tests. The last patient I saw in Beirut came to see me with a large briefcase full of reports from the 51 doctors that she had seen in Cairo, Paris, Jerusalem and Beirut. She was amazed that I did not advise her to be operated on (she had had four operations) and that I advised her to put herself under the care of a Christian Science healer!

Footnotes

1. **Bayard Dodge (1988-1972)**

   The third president of the American University of Beirut (1923-1948). He is credited for translation and editing *The Fihrist of al-Nadîm: A Tenth-Century Survey of Islamic Culture.*

2. **Assadour Aram Altounyan (1857-1950)**

   An Armenian physician born in Turkey. After graduating from the P & S of Columbia in 1885 he went to Germany to work with Dr. Robert Koch. He finally settled in Aleppo, Syria and opened a clinic, which eventually became the finest modern hospital in Syria.

3. **Shukri al-Kowatli (1892-1967)**

   The President of Syria between 1943-1949 and 1955-1958.

Chapter Nineteen

Memorial Hospital

1947 - 1950

The flight home was uneventful, and not very interesting, for we had seen so much and were anxious to get home. Bumps and Jack, who had seen us off, met us. They drove us to Wilton and the ground was covered with snow, the first we had seen on a road since we left. The next day we came back to New York, and after two months of hotel stay, we went to an apartment on East 75th Street, and later to the two lower floors of a house on East 69th Street, opposite the house we had lived in on 68th Street before the hospital moved uptown.

I had decided that it would be the best policy to give up all active surgery when I began my work at the Memorial Hospital in order to avoid any competition with the prima donna attending surgeons. This was wise in many respects, for it gave me an objective attitude in planning certain changes in the organization, which as Clinical Director I was supposed to do, and it made the residents realize that I was not playing any favorites. But I soon realized that my work as Clinical Director would be entirely of an executive nature, although I did see a good many patients in consultation with the attendings and residents. Executive work never appealed to me, and as time went on I found it more and more uninteresting. But I had put my hand to that plough and had to keep it there. However, my relations with the residents continued to be more cordial and constructive, and I had their loyal support in my efforts to improve their responsibilities and in re-organizing some of the departments, such as the record system and the development of the weekly surgical and clinical pathological conferences, which they had not had before. The cooperation of the residents and many of the younger attendings in these changes was enthusiastic, but this was not the case with some of the old die-hards.

I had a great advantage in having the able and constant help of Polly Strong, Arch Strong's widow, whom we had known so many years. She had a fine sense of humor and had the regard and respect of the resident staff, as well as that of most of the attendings. She shielded me from many unnecessary interruptions with great tact and understanding. She was not only an able secretary but also a very good executive, which was what I needed.

My relations with the Presbyterian continued to be most cordial and I saw a great deal of the men there in one way or another. The same was true with the staff of the New York Hospital, for although they were nominally affiliated, the criticism of the former by the latter had been outspoken during the regime of George Heuer [1]. This had created a defense reaction on the part of the Memorial group that prevented any cooperation between the two staffs. Coming from the Presbyterian and having had the best of friendly relations with the New York men, I had an advantage in acting as peacemaker, although with the hazard of a go-between. However, I was able to pave the way for a much better affiliation between the two hospitals, which resulted in advantages to both of them. We organized combined conferences, and opportunities for the residents of the Memorial to use the animal experimental laboratory at the New York until we could build an adequate set-up of our own at the Memorial. That was one of the things I was most anxious to develop, and had made plans for it. The year before I retired from the Memorial, a gift of several hundred thousand dollars together with a grant from the Public Health Service of the Federal Government resulted in the building of one of the most modern and well-equipped experimental laboratories in the country. I insisted that this should be called the laboratory of experimental physiology, and so it was called. For this meant that it would have the support of the scientists in the Sloan-Kettering Institute, which adjoined the Memorial Hospital.

After three years, I felt that I should retire so that a younger man with the experience and training in chemistry and biophysics could succeed me. The man whom I recommended was a former resident of mine at the Presbyterian, and had worked with me in Washington during the war. He had later made a fine reputation at the University of Pennsylvania and at the Yale Medical School, before coming to the Presbyterian as Professor of Surgery with George Humphreys [2]. After several months of negotiations, John Lockwood [3] made the decision to accept our offer. We had several sessions with him and Rhoades as well as with other members of the staff who were very anxious to have him come. He had planned to succeed me on July 1st, 1950, but in the latter part of May of that year he was taken with a severe viral pneumonia and after several weeks of this illness he had a sudden coronary thrombosis and died the next day. This was a dreadful loss, not only to the Memorial, but also to American surgery, for John Lockwood was one of the most promising young surgeons in the country.

This made it necessary for me to stay on another year until we could find the right man to take my place. I took several trips to different parts of the country trying to find the man we wanted. Finally another former resident of mine at the Presbyterian was chosen to take the place of John Lockwood, with whom he had worked. This proved to be a happy and fortunate choice, for Tom Randall [4] has made good in every way and is now able to put through many reforms, some of which I had initiated.

A few weeks before I left, the residents at the Memorial gave me a very genuine and amusing farewell dinner at the university club. Many of the attending staff and some of the trustees also joined the residents. The Toast Master, Guy Robbing, introduced other residents who presented mementoes with apt and amusing quips and sallies. One of the presents that they felt would be useful was a set of larger retractors for the operations that I was planning to do on mice when I moved to Princeton; another was a picture of the Memorial Center with the autographs of the residents and attending. Another (and one that I have worn ever since) was an Omega, self-winding wristwatch, which has kept accurate time and has never been wound. On the reverse side of the gold watch is inscribed, "A.O.Whipple, from the Memorial Staff, 47-51." This was a sendoff that I appreciated deeply, as it was a spontaneous gesture on the part of all the residents.

During the first year at the Memorial I got to know one of the residents quite well, both for his ability as a resident and because he was very much interested in landscape painting. He had worked with Frank Herring [5] in New York two years and had spent his vacation in Burnsville, North Carolina at the Herring-Shorter Painting Class. He told me about this in such glowing terms that Mary and I got intrigued with the idea of going to Burnsville for our vacation the next summer. This started the first of a most delightful three summers in a beautiful part of the mountains of North Carolina with a group of congenial and varied people, all interested in and, for the most part, taking part in the painting class. Two enthusiastic artists, Frank Herring and Edward Shorter, conducted this. The former was a master in both oils and watercolors; the latter was especially interested in oils and portrait work.

Footnotes

1. **George Heuer (1880-1950)**

   Professor of Surgery at the New York Hospital. After completing his training with William Halsted, he established this country's second modern surgical training program outside of Johns Hopkins. It was Heuer who was summoned to operate on the ailing Halsted when he developed cholangitis and gastrointestinal hemorrhage.

2. **George H. Humphreys, II (1903-2001)**

   Chairman of Surgery at the P & S of Columbia University, and Director of Surgical Services at the Presbyterian Hospital (1946-1969).

3. **John S. Lockwood (1907-1950)**

   Born in Shanghai, China, a graduate of Harvard Medical School in 1931. He served as consultant to the Secretary of War in 1942; he then became the Chief of Division of Surgery, serving on the Committee on Medical Research and was a Professor of Surgery at the P & S (1942-1946). He died at the age of 42, two weeks prior to starting his new appointment as Clinical Director and Chief of Surgical Services at the Memorial Hospital.

4. **Henry T. Randall (-1994)**

After his surgical training at the Presbyterian Hospital and service in Europe during World War II, Dr. Randall joined the staff of Sloan-Kettering Hospital in 1951, where he became Chief of Surgical Services and later Vice-president and a Professor of Surgery at Cornell University Medical Center College. In 1967 he moved to Brown University as the surgeon in charge of the division of surgical research at Rhode Island Hospital. Dr. Randall's main interest included metabolism of surgical patients and fluid and electrolytes management.

5. **Frank Stanley Herring (1894-1966)**

A portrait painter born in Pennsylvania and lived in New York City and Milledgeville, Georgia. In New York City he taught at the Grand Central School of Art. In addition to the High Museum of Art, Atlanta, Georgia, his works are to be seen at the collection of Georgia State College for Women in Milledgeville, and the Mecklenburg Court House, Charlotte, North Carolina.

Chapter Twenty

Princeton, hobbies, honors and final years

1951 - 1963

One of the problems facing us when I decided to retire from the Memorial and New York, was where to go and where to settle for the rest of our days. When we had returned from Beirut we had considered the possibility of living in Princeton, where we had wanted to retire, but the fact that there was a great housing shortage there at the time and the fact that I had to be at the Memorial before nine in the morning, soon convinced us that we would have to continue to live in New York. But the idea of living in Princeton with all its associations and attractions stayed uppermost in our minds.

In the spring of 1951 when we were beginning to settle our affairs on East 69th Street, we came to Princeton and had a talk with George Brakeley [1], the Vice-president and Treasurer of the university. He said we should apply to the Stanworth Apartments, but said that they had a long waiting list and that he would do what he could to get us an apartment if there were one vacant. Meanwhile one of my classmates, Lou Conklin, asked me to have lunch with him at the Ritz-Carleton to talk over my plans. When I told him I was anxious to resume a piece of research on the circulation of the spleen that David DeKenzie and I had started ten years previously, but which had been interrupted by the war, he was very understanding and said he would like to make a contribution to such a piece of research. He sent me a check for $5,000, which was to be used in the Biological Laboratory in Princeton for that research. This was a most unexpected and welcome windfall that settled my resolve to reside in Princeton.

A short time after this check arrived, President Harold Dodd [2] spoke to me after a meeting of the Executive Committee of the Trustees of Princeton. He said he had heard that we were considering coming to Princeton, and asked me if I would be willing to act as adviser to the pre-medical students in the university, a much needed service. This appealed to me greatly, for I knew about some of the problems of this group of students and their need for sound advice during their four years in the university. I also told him about the gift that my classmate had made to the Biological Laboratory. He immediately said that he would take the matter up with Arthur Parpart, the Head of the Department, and would see that every facility would be available to me.

The next week I had a message from Prof. Parpart asking me to come to Princeton to discuss my project. After a very pleasant talk with him, he said that the study of the blood had always interested him and that he would welcome my working in his laboratory. Knowing this, I asked him if he would be willing to work on my project with me, and share in the publication of anything that might come out of it. This he said he would be glad to do. This meant more than I had hoped for, because he is a great experimental physiologist and has a complete and efficient machine shop where they can turn out any kind of gadget, and I knew we would have to have special ones made for this study.

Three weeks before we were to leave for Burnsville, we were notified that one of the apartments in Stanworth would be available if we wanted it. Mum and I came down and looked it over and immediately took it, with the understanding that we could move into it in September after we had returned from Seecelo. In the meantime we had stored our belongings in the Lincoln warehouse in New York and had other things stored in the barn in Wilton. These combined were a total accumulation of years of collecting that we knew we could never move to any apartment in Princeton. As I said in a speech at the dinner that my residents gave us in New York, "At one time we had four houses with lots of room, but no time; now we have four rooms with no space, but plenty of time."

To retire from an active surgical career without interesting things to do, and to retire with congenial hobbies and avocations are two very different concepts of entering the sunset of life. During the war, while I was in London, I spent some of my spare time in the British Museum, following my interest in the study of the role of the Nestorians in their link between the Greeks and the Arabs in medical history. One day I came across an anonymous saying that has stayed with me ever since. It read, "The ability to decorate the idle hour is the proof and measure of one's capacity to live." It should have added, "in retirement." There is no agreement about the decoration, but that is where the wide choice comes in for the individual.

This brings up the subject of hobbies and avocations. I have had too many perhaps and, like the Jack-of-All-Trades, I have been master of none. But it has been pleasant and interesting. In enumerating them, you will see that I have too many. As a result of having lived in the Middle East and later in the various parts of the Near East, I became infected with the lure of the Orient early on. My father introduced me to the lure of Persian rugs and oriental antiques, for that was one of his bodies. The dallals, itinerant dealers in these goods, discovered father's interest and used to be regular callers on him, showing him good, bad, and indifferent examples of their wares. He was a connoisseur, and their efforts to foist fakes or shoddy specimens on him were unsuccessful. As a result, over the years that he lived in Tabriz he collected an unusually fine lot of Greek, Parthian and Sassanian coins, as well as fine examples of Persian art and some fine specimens of Persian and Caucasian rugs.

I remember well the day he called me into his study on my tenth birthday. He showed me a beautiful Farahan rug, 9 by 5 feet, which he said he had just purchased at a great bargain for ten Tomans, the equivalent of $12. He asked me what I thought of it. I told him at once that I thought it was one of the finest that I had ever seen. He said. "Well, if you like it, I am going to give it to you with the understanding that you will take the best care of it, and that you will leave it for your son and grandson." This was indeed a surprise and a gift that I have always cherished, and I have kept it in as good a condition as the intervening seventy years have permitted. It is still a very fine rug, though somewhat worn. In New York I was once offered $440 for it, but of course, would not sell it at any price. It has been in my study ever since I began to practice. I plan to leave it to my son and then to my grandson, as my father asked me to do.

This interest in Persian and oriental rugs has stayed with me, although I have not been able to purchase as many as I have wanted. But it has been a source of many intriguing visits to the auctions in New York and the Armenian and Levantine rug dealers in that city, usually accompanied by mum who has become quite a connoisseur and discriminating in her taste for these articles. But at first I had a time with her when we went to one of the Armenian places, for she would spot a fine rug that appealed to her and let the dealer know it. This of course was nuts to the oriental scrooge, for he would immediately hike the price. I had to explain to her that the way to approach these orientals was to examine a number of rugs that you are not interested in, and casually look at the one you wanted. After asking the price of others, including the one you wanted, you would begin to offer a price far below the one asked. This made the oriental realize that he was dealing with someone who knew oriental methods and the tricks of the trade. Very often I would inform the dealer that he was wrong about the make of the rug. This resulted in an argument until I told him that I had lived in Persia and was not a fool when it came to spotting the kinds and prices of his wares.

My interest in things oriental has resulted in my acquiring a fair number of books on various phases of the subject. One of my prizes is a first edition of *The Adventures of Hajji Baba*, a first fascinating and accurate account of the adventures of a Persian freelance. It was supposed to have been written by a Persian, but was actually written by Du Maurier, an English diplomat, and for many years it remained a literary hoax. Because of Du Maurier's long stay in Persia, he knew the life and manners of the Persians of the 18th century so well that his story had every sign of having been written by a native. Because of the lack of room for bookshelves in the apartments we have lived in, I decided to give my collection of books on Persian art to the university library, where I can consult any of the volumes whenever I want.

Among the books that I have kept are a few that I had as a small boy in Persia - copybooks and text books in Persian and French. One of them is a copy of the *Gulistan* by the poet Saadi. This is a collection of stories and poems that I can still read because I knew many of them by heart when I studied Persian in Tabriz and Oroomiah. Saadi was the great storywriter and poet of the 13th century. His admirers visit his tomb in Shiraz every day. An example of the kind of story written by him and appealing to the people who admired a ruler interested in the welfare of his citizens is as follows:

"They tell about Nushirwan the Just (a Sassanian King of Persia) who was on a hunting expedition. On the hunting field they were roasting the game for the King. But it was discovered that no salt had been brought with them. A slave was ordered to get some salt from a nearby village. Nushirvan said 'be sure you get the salt at a price so that a bad custom be not established and the village be not ruined.' They said, 'What loss could come from such a trifle?' The King replied, 'The origin of tyranny in the world was small at first; others have added to it 'till it has reached its present state.' Then follow two couplets; if the King were to eat an apple from the orchard of a subject without pay, his followers would pluck up the tree by the roots. For five eggs which the sultan might deem lawful plunder, his army would roast a thousand fowls on spits."

The collection of coins that I have mentioned was doing little good in the apartment, so mum and I decided to give it to the Department of Oriental Studies in the university, where it might be of some help to the students who study the history of the Near and Middle East. Since then, one of the students has used them in preparing his Ph.D. thesis.

A hobby, which I followed when we moved into the old house in Wilton, was carpentry. Because I had learned some of that occupation when I lived in Oroomiah, with Eli Allen, I got interested in making some of the furniture for the house which we had bought unfurnished; this applied especially to tables, four of the stretcher type and one a butterfly table which I copied from a photograph and measurements of an old New England butterfly table. This and the first stretcher table, modeled after a Wallace Nutting antique of 1680, we gave to Sis. She kept them both in perfect condition.

Enough has been said about the cello as a hobby. The fact that I found it hard to practice surgery and the cello account for my being such a poor amateur at the latter. But I got a great deal of pleasure out of it, although I am sure mum must have spent many an uncomfortable hour listening to me practice. But coming to know Bedrich Vaska and the good times that we had with the scrub quartet was compensation enough. Perhaps the most worthwhile thing about it was that it gave me an appreciation for the artistry of stringed instrument playing that I could never have had if I had not struggled with the cello. And of course the musical atmosphere that we had in Persia, Duluth, and Oberlin had much to do with my love of music.

As regards painting as a hobby, there is no doubt in my mind that landscape and portrait work is the most absorbing occupation, even more so than music. For that reason it is a very good thing for a doctor, as an escape from his many pressing problems. Furthermore, it does not require the constant practice to do something worthwhile, and it can be pursued at odd times and during vacations much more easily. Also the brushes and paint box can be carried about with less effort than required by a cello or piano.

The start that Frank Chase gave me was most helpful, for he did not take my efforts too seriously and interlaced his lessons with delightful times on the golf course in Nantucket. He was such a good companion and could take part in any gathering, with amusing stories about himself and his friends. He was a favorite with the natives of Nantucket as well as with the off-islanders. Unfortunately, several years ago his eyesight and his ability to walk any distance made him gave up his work as a painter and teacher, and death was a kind release for him.

As a beginner, I was taught the difference between an artistic composition and a photographic picture. Like so many beginners, I tried to put leaves on the trees and did not use the artistic license of outing things in the picture and leaving out others. Frank was a master in portraying trees in different settings and in different seasons, and was a master in painting clouds, which gave a real individuality to his landscapes.

Comparing Frank Chase with Frank Herring and Edward Shorter is somewhat difficult. They were all devoted teachers and each had his own style. In oil landscape work, Frank Chase was ablest and most original, but in watercolors, Frank Herring was in a class by himself. Some of the portraits that he made in that medium were really remarkable. One of these that I especially remember was that of a former slave in North Carolina, done when she was at the ripe old age of 105. She had innumerable wrinkles in her face and was the perfect picture of relaxation in her pose as she sat in her old rocking chair. Frank Herring was also remarkable in the rapidity with which he worked. In his demonstrations of portrait work in oils or watercolors he would finish a portrait in less than two hours. At one of these demonstrations his model did not appear, so he asked me to pose for him. This was an interesting experience, which we duplicated the next year when he asked me to sit for a portrait in oils. This time he took four sessions to do it. But mum and others thought that the quickie that he had done the year before was a better likeness. Both mum and I sat as models for the portrait class. A sketch of me, which one of the talented young artists did in charcoal, was considered a very good portrait of me, and mum had it enlarged. But I always said that if I had had a crucifix in my hand, I could have been taken for a pope. Of another portrait of me I shall have more to say later.

The study of medical history may be called a hobby if one does not make a vocation of it. Medical history differs from that of other subjects in that it deals with the profession if one is a doctor, and for that reason, is more interesting to physicians than to lay readers. One of the revealing aspects of the study is the effect that certain periods of non-medical history had in advancing or retarding the progress of medicine. The prejudice that the ancients had against dissection and post-mortem examinations was continued through the Middle Ages, as shown by the Papal Bull that read, "Ecclesia abhorret a sanguine" meaning the Church shuns blood. This did not encourage surgery, and that branch of therapy was delegated to the barbers that lived in the monasteries for the purpose of shaving the faces and tonsures of the monks. In the Dark Ages, the monks were, for the most part, the physicians who treated the ills of the natives with prayers and incantations, urging the sick to accept their infirmities as the will of God. But they would have nothing to do with anything like injuries or shedding of blood; this was delegated to the barbers. They became known as barber-surgeons and wore short tunics whereas the monks wore long cassoks. They were called the long-robed and the barbers, the short-robed. Even up to the end of the 17th century, the surgeons who had given up their work as barbers were still called barber-surgeons. In England today the surgeon is addressed as "Mister", while the physician is called "Doctor".

Another interesting feature of the study of medical history is finding how close some of the physicians and scientists were to the discovery of basic facts that have made medicine what it is today, and what difficulty the men who made great discoveries had in convincing the profession of their validity. This was certainly true in the demonstration of the principles of antisepsis and asepsis, and in the proof that bacteria were the cause of infection.

One of the reasons why I became interested in one period of medical history was because it had to do with the old Christian sect of the Nestorians, for I had lived among these people in Oroomiah and our servants in Tabriz were Nestorians. I had learned to read their language, the Syriac, and to speak it when I was ten years old. I became intrigued with their role as the connecting link between Greek and Arabic medicine, and I had studied original sources on the subject in Latin, French, and Syriac writings in the British Museum and the Vatican libraries during my different trips abroad. Besides this period, I had read a number of texts on the history of medicine and have several of them in my library. One of the most revealing books on the subject of surgery during the middle of the 18th century is a diary written by a young surgeon, telling of his experiences in one of the leading hospitals in London as a medical student, and later as a surgeon on-board one of the

British warships. This describes, startlingly and starkly, the kind of surgery that was done in those days, without benefit of anesthesia or asepsis. Anyone coming to the hospital with a compound fracture had an immediate amputation of the extremity of the fracture. The hospital mortality rate with these operations was well over 60 per cent.

Writing may or may not be a hobby. I have had to do a great deal of it, but most of it has had to do with surgical subjects. It has been an interesting experience and, by and large, I have enjoyed it. Over the years of my surgical work I have written some 170 articles or papers, many of which were read at surgical meetings, and others were sent to surgical journals as well as to medical journals. Those that were read at surgical meetings and later published in periodicals were a heterogeneous lot, some of them much better than others. The one presented before such a society as the American Association had to be most carefully prepared, and had to do with the work at the Presbyterian Hospital and the College of P & S. This means that it provided an opportunity to travel to various cities and medical schools, as well as the chance to see the work of my surgical friends in other clinics. This was one of the most pleasant experiences. Among old friends, seen in their homes and in their operating rooms, there were no miracles, and one was able to get the "low down" on many false rumors. The exchanges of experiences and of points of view were rewards of these visits and meetings. This was especially true of the meetings of the travel clubs, like the Society of Clinical Surgery and the Interurban Surgical, the membership of which was made up of heads of surgical departments in the country.

But not all of my papers were surgical in nature. The few that I prepared on the history of medicine were published in the *Annals of the History of Medicine*. Others on non-medical subjects were read at the Charaka Club [3]. This is a delightful club that has been active for the last 75 years. It was started by a group of men, physicians, like Sir William Osler, Harvey Cushing, Bernard Sachs and Charles Dana. It was organized for the purpose of presenting non-medical subjects and hobbies of the members who were all physicians. The membership has been an interesting one over the years, and the insistence of keeping "shop talk" out of the proceedings has been attractive. Some ten volumes of these proceedings have been published. I have been a member for about 30 years. The meetings are held at the Coffee House in New York five times a year, and are preceded by a very good dinner.

Some of the papers that were read by other members of the club I remember especially well and were entitled: "The Problem of the Professional Guinea Pig," by Osler Abbott; "What is Time?" by Carl Vogel, an authority on clocks and timepieces; "The Vagaries of the Vivisectionist, turned Surgeon," by Sam Lambert; "Doctors and Gardens," by Frederick Peterson; "A Meeting with Robert Browning," by Bernard Sachs, and the "The Substance of Dreams," by Foster Kennedy. Some of the papers that I read at the club were: "The Cedars of Lebanon - Their Cause of the Many Invasions of the Lebanon"; "The Role of the Nestorians as the Connecting Link between Greek and Arabic Medicine"; "Hours Spent in the Vatican Library"; "The Adventures of Hajji Baba, a Delightful Literary Hoax"; "Ramblings of a Rug Addict", and "An Account of a Recent Trip to North Africa". The majority of the members were also members of the Century Club, so that I knew most of them as old friends.

This brings me to the account of my experiences in the Century [4]. This is one of the oldest and most select clubs in New York. It has always been considered a unique and distinguished association. It was organized more than a century ago. To belong to it, one must be an amateur (the definition of just what that means is not too clear, even to the members), but he must have an interesting avocation or hobby. No account of wealth means anything but a handicap for one's election to membership, so there are only a few millionaires in that class. Most of the members are in one of the professions or are artists of a kind: painters, sculptors, writers or musicians. Every year they hold an exhibit of the professional painters' work, and another for the amateur painters, in the art gallery.

During the last thirty years of my membership, I have come to know and cherish the friendship of painters, sculptors, musicians, doctors, lawyers, writers and "amateurs" whom I never would have known but for the Century Association. The monthly dinner of the members, held every first Thursday of the month, is a very enjoyable affair where one sees so many of his friends and comes to know new members. The large long table (it is oval) has a fine tradition. When a member takes his place at the table he may be sitting next to a member from out of town, whom he has never met. He does not wait for an introduction, but enters into conversation with his neighbor as if he had always known him. In this way I have had some of the most interesting talks with men whom I had never met before, and some of them I have never met again - interesting ships that pass in the night.

Some of my most delightful and whimsical friends are Centurians of long-standing. The trouble is that too often they are added to the list of the deceased in the Year Book, for most of the members are in the upper age brackets. Serving on one of the committees of the club is always an experience, especially on the Committee on Admissions, which I did for three years, as well as on the Board of Trustees. Because of the large membership of writers and literary-minded, the library is unusually fine and contains many autographed first editions by members of the club.

Another very worthwhile and distinguished group of which I have had the privilege of belonging is the Board of Trustees of Princeton University. This is not a club, but has many of the qualities of a select group. It is made up of what are called charter trustees, elected by the Board, and alumni trustees, chosen by ballot from the alumni to represent them in different parts of the country. I was a charter trustee for nine years and have been an emeritus trustee since 1952. I have sat on different boards in the past but this one is unique in that every member has a definite duty and is held responsible for making good on it. Harold Dodd was the President of the university for twenty years and had a great deal to do with creating a spirit of loyalty and cooperation among all the members of the Board, encouraging all of them to take an active part in the discussions and in determining the policies of the Board. Until I retired at the age of 70, the rule of the Board, I was Chairman of the Committee on Health of the students, and reported twice a year on the health problems. When a trustee retires he is expected to attend the meetings of the Board, but does not have any active duties or a vote in the meetings. Living in Princeton made my attendance at the meeting easy and enjoyable when I did not have any definite assignments.

Another hobby that I followed for some time was the collecting and studying of the hands of surgeons and physicians. At first I had the idea that there would be a definite difference in the shape and make-up of the hands of the two groups of practitioners. But as I collected models of some eighty hands of well-known surgeons whom I had known in the American Surgical Association, and some thirty internists' hands, I realized that there were no differences. It soon became evident that, as in all walks of life, character was often expressed in the hand. Some interesting examples of this were shown in the hands of doctors with strong or striking personalities. Harvey Cushing [5], who was always positive in his opinions and well aware of his importance, sent me his hand, cast in bronze, with all his fingers in full extension and with all the tendons on the back of his hand tense and showing. Rudolph Matas [6] of New Orleans, a most modest and cultured gentleman, always known for his desire to give his friends and associates full credit for everything that they had done (which resulted in his reading papers of interminable length) sent me the cast of his hand that suggested more than anything else a frightened bird seeking its nest.

The men of artistic temperament, whether surgeons or physicians, had very much the same type of hands, with slender finders longer than average. Most of the surgeons, because of their use of surgical instruments over long periods of time, had thicker and stronger palms and inter-osseous muscles than the internists. This was to be expected. This collection of hands stood, on the top of my bookshelves in my office at the Presbyterian for several years and, when I retired, I left the collection to the surgical department. But, like all collections that are not interesting to the donee, as they are to the donor, I am sure the hands will in time disappear in the limbo of the forgotten. At any rate I had fun collecting them and studying them, and it was for me a hobby, but not for anyone else.

Games may be hobbies. I have had three, none of which I took seriously enough to play well, but which gave me a lot of pleasure. I first took up golf in Evasion, Illinois, in 1903, when I was tutoring one of my classmates. After we had lived in New York for several years, I began playing again in a desultory way, with some of the men at the Presbyterian: Jim Corscaden, Alphonse Dochez, Fred Sancroft and Warfield Longcope. This was on an old course in Flushing, before any of us owned cars, and the trolley trip to Flushing was not exciting. Later, when we spent the summers in Wilton, I used to play with some of the Wilton and Ridgefield people on the fine Silver Springs course. But the golf club I enjoyed the most was St. Andrews in Hastings, not far from Riverdale, New York. The atmosphere there was rather unique in that there were no cliques and one could always get a match, or join a foursome, the handicaps making the game fairly even. Many of the men that I knew there were members of the Century as well, so that we knew each other from two angles. The course is one of the oldest in the country and has some interesting holes that can penalize poor shots.

Golf possesses the advantages of fresh air and good companionship in the exercise that it gives. The one thing the golfer should avoid, good or bad, is taking the game too seriously. I have seen several players who got so angry at their game that they got no pleasure out of it and finally gave it up, for that reason. But, like boxing, it is good discipline and the control of one's temper pays good dividends. This I saw especially on the old course in Nantucket, for if one had to look for his ball in the sand dunes, the temper gets hotter than the sand. I should have mentioned this course as one that gave the boys and I many of our happiest days. I believe I spoke of the two holes on that course that I aced, and then within a period of two days. Since then I never came within feet of doing it again.

Another game that in later years I have especially enjoyed is cowboy pool. This is a Century Club tradition, and is not as well known as other forms of pool and billiards. It is a very happy combination of both, and is best played as a foursome. At the Century the handicaps are so well recorded on a board that it gives individuals playing the game an equal chance. The game is not won until the last ball - a white one - is caromed off the table into one of the six pockets. The reason I have enjoyed playing the game or watching it, is that it is played in the basement of the club where almost every day after five o'clock, genial addicts of the game can be found at one or more of the five tables. Here all semblance of dignity is abandoned, and the noise of the shouts of glee over a difficult shot, or the laments of the man who has missed an easy one, can be heard well beyond the basement. This basement is the meeting ground of not only those who are playing pool or billiards, but of other members who come down just to hear the fun and watch the antics of the addicts. Artists, sculptors, writers, musicians, lawyers, doctors are all represented by the best of them. Certainly some of my closest friendships in the Century were made there and continued as the result of our meetings in the basement.

Chess is, of course, the oldest and the most difficult of games. It apparently was invented in India and was introduced into Persia in the 8th century. It was introduced into Europe by the Crusaders, and became the favorite game of the cardinals; some of the moves are named after them. It is a game absolutely devoid of chance or luck. One wins or loses the game depending upon whether he makes mistakes and his opponent takes advantage of them, or vice versa. It is again a mistake to take this game too seriously, for it is easy to develop an insomnia in thinking over the moves, and more than one professional chess master has gone insane with it, especially if he has been playing ten or more games blindfolded.

Chess is the most universal game in the world for it is played in all the civilized countries, and in some of the less civilized ones. It is especially popular in the Latin and Slavic nations. One sees it played on the ocean liners for it is a good way to pass the time. On more than one occasion I have played the game with a man who could not speak English and I could not speak his language, but one does not need a spoken tongue to play chess, for the rules are now universal.

But I have spent too much time discussing the subject of hobbies; if one has them, he is sure to discuss them. The preceding pages will show that both mum and I had plenty to occupy our time during retirement. She loved to sew and knit as well as read, and came to know some of our neighbors so well that they visited her at the expense of some of the things she wanted to do. The occupations that I have had, have not been burdened with the responsibility and anxiety that always accompanied my work as an operating surgeon. Nor have the days been disciplined by the regular hours and the duties of a routine schedule as in the forty years of hospital work. Freedom from the many committee meetings that I had to attend (heaven has been described as a place where there are no committee meetings), has been a blessing in itself.

Among other things, I have had time to read many books that I have wanted to and have enjoyed the privileges of the Princeton Library, or the Firestone, as it is called. It is the most interesting university library in the country, for it is built for study and designed for the use of the students; it is essentially a functional structure. One is allowed to go through the stacks, the lighting is good and the building is air-conditioned with many small lounges and tables as well as 500 carels, or cubicles, used mostly by the seniors in writing their theses.

I should have said that in the spring of 1952 I was asked to take part in the centenary of William S. Halsted, the first Professor of Surgery at the Johns Hopkins Medical School and Hospital. The title of my address at that meeting was "Halsted's New York Period." I had always been a great admirer of Halsted and had been especially interested in his career in New York and the circumstances that led to his leaving New York to go to Baltimore. The committee that had charge of the program accepted my suggested title, in as much as all the other papers describing Halsted's career had to do with his life and work in Baltimore.

The celebration of the centenary was well planned, and the elaborate program was well carried out. Ned and Agnes Park had asked mum and I to stay with them during the program, and Ned had been asked to introduce me at the dinner when Leriche of Paris and I were after-dinner speakers. At the dinner, which was attended by the members of the Society of Clinical Surgery and the Society of University Surgeons, as well as by all the Hopkins faculty and Halsted's many friends and admirers in and out of Baltimore (some 250 men and women in all), Ned Park gave me a very amusing and flattering introduction. My good friend Alfred Blalock [7], the Professor of Surgery at the Hopkins, was the Toast Master. The address that I gave was before a very sympathetic audience, and I had many letters of appreciation after we returned to Princeton. Attending the Halsted centenary were a number of my former residents. They met after the dinner and had a talkfest that lasted until two o'clock the next morning. They decided that it was time my former residents and interns did something worthwhile as a tribute to me as their teacher and guide during their surgical training. This meeting resulted in their appointing a committee of five of my former residents and associates at the Presbyterian: Henry Cooper, Pat Elliott, Dave MacKenzie, Grant Sanger and Ed Self, to arrange to have my portrait done and to have it presented to the Presbyterian Hospital at a dinner to be given later in the fall.

Before I knew anything about this, the committee had sent letters to 217 men and women who had served under me while I was Professor of Surgery at the Columbia-Presbyterian Medical Center. The response was so much greater than the committee had expected that they decided to have the amount of money beyond the expenses, of having the portrait painted and that of the dinner, given to Princeton University for me to carry on my research work in the Biological Laboratory.

The next fall I was asked to come to the University of Chicago to take part in the celebration of the 25th anniversary of the founding of the University of Chicago Medical School. There I spent three very interesting days and, with four other men, was given the honorary degree of Doctor of Science. The other men were Anton Carlson, the eminent physiologist of the university, James Gamble, the well-known pediatrician of Boston, Tibbett, Professor of Medicine at New York University, and George Whipple [8], Dean and Professor of Pathology at the University of Rochester Medical School. I had known all of these men and had worthwhile talks with them during the days of the meeting. George Whipple and I marched together in the academic procession. He said, as we were approaching the Chapel where the degrees were to be conferred. "Allen, we can be sure that the two Whipples never marched together before to be given the degree of Doctor of Science at the same time." I agreed with him. For many years we had agreed that we were cousins, but never investigated how far removed the relationship was. Both he and I had the other's mail sent to us; mine dealt with some pancreatic problems, his, with some liver or blood problem, for he had shared in the Nobel Prize for the discoveries that were made in the role of the liver in treating anemias.

Medical and surgical societies and academies have had medals and lectureships endowed and named. These, for one reason or other, have to be awarded to individuals periodically. They are usually given to individuals who have served for a long time or have retired after what is considered a special accomplishment or contribution to medical science and practice. In the course of many years, a number of such awards have come to me, some of them deserved and greatly appreciated. For a number of these occasions it meant traveling to cities and medical centers a long way from home, and in some instances, mum's and my expenses were paid for the trip.

The award that I especially prize was the Bigelow Medal given to me by the Boston Surgical Society in 1941. This award has been given only eight times before to men like Will Mayo [9], Rudolph Matas, John Finney [10] and Harvey Cushing. What I appreciated especially was the presentation of the large gold medal by my great friend, David Cheever [11], with the following words, "Dr. Whipple, having voted to confer on you the Bigelow Medal, the Boston Surgical Society has delegated to me the honor of presenting it to you. We, the members of the Society, and others of your friends here assembled, including many of the Fellows of the American College of Surgeons who are attending their annual meeting in this city, need no enlightenment about the reasons for this award; but citizens in other walks of life will wish to know the grounds for the bestowal of so signal an honor - an honor paid to but eight other recipients in the twenty-six years since the medal was established. A brief citation of these grounds is therefore appropriate.

"Born in Persia where you spent, the formative years of childhood and boyhood, you were nevertheless not imbued with the fatalist and mystical philosophies of the Orient, but found rather the master key to life's problems in the principle of free will and self-determination bequeathed to you from seven generations of your New England ancestors.

"At Princeton you received your cultural and basic scientific education, and it is an interesting example of the shrewd intuition of youth that your classmates voted you the man most likely to succeed in later life. Your medical degree was won from the College of Physicians and Surgeons of Columbia University, and there followed internships at the Roosevelt and Sloane Maternity Hospitals. You then entered the service of the Presbyterian Hospital as surgeon and pathologist, passing rapidly up the steps of surgical preferment, until, in 1921, but thirteen years after graduating from medical school, you were appointed Professor of Surgery at Columbia University and Director of Surgery at the Presbyterian Hospital. Your post bears the name of the illustrious Valentine Mott, who, a century ago was your predecessor as Professor of Surgery and the leading surgeon in the greatest city in the country.

"The qualities you have displayed in this high post and the things you have accomplished must be touched upon, although at the certain risk of offending your modest self-appraisal. As a surgeon, you have accomplished much and you have even advanced the science and perfected the art; nothing in the whole field has been alien to your interest. To whatever problem you have addressed yourself you have brought clarification. Whatever tissue or organ is to be the object of your beneficent attention, your procedures are based on thorough knowledge of its anatomy, its physiology, and its pathology. The diseases of the upper abdomen have constituted one of your special interests. You have demonstrated convincingly the possibility of the successful extirpation of the duodenum and the head of the pancreas for carcinoma; your success in the diagnosis and removal of pancreatic tumors for the cure of that distressing and fatal malady, with hyperinsulinism makes you the leading authority in that field; on the physiology and pathology of the spleen - described by Galen as 'an organ full of mystery', you have thrown light that has helped to establish a rational approach to surgical therapies. Indeed, your most recent research has, by ingenious methods, perhaps definitely settled the old problem of the nature of the circulation in the spleen and portal bed. Your common sense has told you that the profundity of knowledge alone on the surgeon's part will not ensure a successful operation, that the successful technical application of the knowledge to human tissues is of equal value; therefore you have found not unworthy of intensive study the everyday problem of suture and ligature material and of wound healing.

"For twenty years you have directed the surgical service of the Presbyterian Hospital and the teaching of surgery in the college of Physicians and Surgeons. This has been a period of change of plans, in organization, in methods, in social outlook, when failure might have been the administration of one who had not your courage, your gentleness, your practical idealism, your fairness, and, above all, your intellectual integrity. You might have inspired the ancient aphorism: *Fortiter in re, suaviter in modo.* Doubtless you have found your greatest satisfaction in the relief of human ills but scarcely less have been your happiness in the education of young men - you are a crusader for better training in surgery, in both undergraduate and postgraduate years. Distinguished as a clinician you have led by your investigative point of view beyond the clinic to fruitful study in the laboratory. In inspiring research you have been a veritable catalyst - although perhaps the analogy is not a sound one, since a catalyst, in achieving its reactions, does not spend itself.

"A full Curriculum Vitae vestrae should list the hundred titles from your pen under which you have shared your knowledge with your colleagues, should enumerate the societies in which you hold membership and high office, should report honors, and should speak of your help in creating and supporting high standards of surgical work. It should mention the talents in music, in painting, the interest in books and history, which adds to your Spartan qualities of courage and self-discipline, attributes more Attic in their nature. It may only hint at tender personal relationships, which through the years have supported you by your hearthstone.

"Among your many avocations, I am told, is numismatics. Here then is a medal to add to your collection, beautifully wrought in purest gold. It is indeed a jewel to be treasured, but it is our happy belief that it will chiefly signify to you an enduring token of the confidence and affection of fellow workers in the field of surgery."

There were other occasions when I was invited to give named lectures and to receive medals or awards, and the one that I especially prize was the Evarts A. Graham Medal and Lectureship, established in honor of my old friend and classmate. Mum and I were guests in the Graham home and had a delightful visit with them. In the same week I was given the honorary decree of Doctor of Science by Washington University at their commencement where both Evarts and Helen were on the faculty.

A medal which I have never prized or shown, was sent me by Adolph Hitler for taking care of four of the officers that were so badly burned at the time of the explosion of the Hindenburg [12]. This medal had the Iron Cross on it. One of the instructions that we had from Berlin at that time was to be sure not to give any Jewish blood in transfusing the four officers. We had already used several pints from the mixed blood bank and this had much to do with saving the lives of the four men.

During the first four years of retirement in Princeton much of my time was taken up in the following occupations: the work in the Biological Laboratory with Professor Parpart and Joseph Chang, a Korean postgraduate, in the study of the circulation of the blood in the spleen of the living mouse and bat; acting as adviser to the pre-medical students in the university; weekly visits to the Bronx and the East Orange Veterans' Hospitals as senior consultant in surgery; planting and weeding the three flower beds around our apartment; and lastly, with work on the Board of Trustees of the American University of Beirut and the Iran Foundation in New York.

Of the latter, a few words of explanation are necessary. Mohammed Nemazee, a native of the city of Shiraz in Iran, left his native city to come to America. He was educated in a Seventh Day Adventist College and then left for Hong Kong, China, where he engaged in the China Trade, built a shipping fleet and made a fortune. He returned to Washington and decided to do something worthwhile for his native city of Shiraz. What was needed most was a pure water supply, for the people had been using the water that ran through the jubes, or water courses, along the streets as a source of water for drinking, washing and every other purpose. This had for centuries caused outbreaks of typhoid and dysentery in the inhabitants. Nemazee spent over four million dollars in digging artesian wells and piping water to the homes of those who could pay for it, and setting up water siphons in the public squares so that the poor could draw the water for drinking purposes. Within three years the undertakers of the city complained to the mayor that the water works were ruining their business!

Nemazee then decided that the city needed a modern hospital. Not knowing anything about hospitals, he decided to get advice from qualified sources. Having heard that I had lived in Iran and was the Professor of Surgery at Columbia, he came to me with Dr. Torab Mehra, and asked me to serve as a chairman of an advisory committee to guide him in his plans to build a hospital in Shiraz along the best American methods. He wisely said that he wanted it to be a training ground for Iranian doctors. We had a most interesting conference with him and Dr. Mehra, a graduate of the Long Island Medical College and the Johns Hopkins School of Public Health, who was to be the director of the hospital when it was built. I organized a committee of seven doctors from the hospitals in New York and the Rockefeller Foundation, and for three years we planned and blue-printed a hospital for two hundred beds, and got the hospital built. The iron framework and all of the equipment had to come from this country and there were annoying delays, but by 1953 it was finished enough that the American doctors whom we were able to get to start the several services were in Shiraz and eager to get the hospital working. The Chief of Surgery was Bob Hiatt, a former resident of mine at the Presbyterian; the Chief of Medicine was from the University Hospital in New Haven; the pathologist was an able colored doctor from one of the colored hospitals in the south.

I had to make two visits to Shiraz, to settle some problems, and I assisted Bob Hiatt in the first operation that was done in the new hospital. He repaired a hernia on the father of Dr. Mehra. We had an all-Presbyterian team at that first operation, including the anesthetist and the operating room nurse.

At the dedication of the hospital in 1955, the Shah and his Queen took the leading part, and within six years the hospital, called the Nemazee Hospital, was by far the finest and best staffed in the Middle East. Dr. Mehra has done an amazing job in organizing and keeping the hospital up-to-date and carrying out the purpose of the donor. Nemazee has spent more than five million dollars in the building and equipment. He has almost always accepted the advice of the advisory committee. I remember at one of the earlier meetings we said that the summer in Shiraz would be very hard for the American doctors. He said, "I will put up twenty air-conditioned houses for them," and he did.

With the development of the hospital, a training school for nurses was started and it was the first one staffed with capable American nursing instructors. At first we were concerned about the possibility of getting qualified Iranian young women to take up the training for nursing. The ancient prejudice of having a woman having anything to do with the care of men, and the old dread of coming in touch with the dead were the two reasons for the fear we had, that few women would take up nursing. But after the first year the number of candidates began to increase, so that after ten years the number of applicants was far greater than the number of young Iranian women who were admitted for training. This was an unexpected result.

The organization of the hospital and staff was, as expected, faced with problems and difficulties and delays. These were discouraging to the people who had been appointed and had gone out to Shiraz. This became critical and threatened the success of the project, so that the Iran Foundation, which by that time had taken over the management of the hospital, asked me to go to Shiraz to report on the situation and to try to resolve some of the difficulties.

Mum, as always, told me it was my duty to go, and said she would go to the Bings in Birmingham while I was away. So in November I left for Iran flying by way of Paris, Rome and Beirut to reach Teheran. I am including excerpts from a diary that I kept on my way to and from Iran.

"November 2nd, 1954. I am on a Pan-American plane over the Atlantic. It has been a hectic four days since I decided to go to Shiraz. This meant getting a new passport, another vaccination, canceling a number of appointments, arranging transportation for mum, and collecting data for my mission to the hospital in Shiraz. I arrived in the Orly airport the next day, and after an hour, left for Rome, stopping in Geneva where the transients were herded into a special room where Swiss watches of all makes were exhibited to tempt the travelers. I arrived in Rome at 9 o'clock at a much larger, but disorganized airport. The two suitcases that had been sent on from New York were not to be found, but as the plane was on its way to Bombay and Calcutta, I had vision of my bags landing in India. Finally an Italian stewardess appeared from nowhere to tell me that the suitcases were at the customs counter and that the Scandinavian plane that I was supposed to take to Teheran did not have room for me, so that I was supposed to take a K.L.M. plane two days later. If this had to be, I was glad it had to be in the Eternal City where there were so many favorite haunts to re-visit. A taxi took me to the Hassler Hotel where a room had been reserved for me.

"November 4th. The many matin bells wakened me at an early hour. After a cafe complet, I went to the K.L.M. office to be told that my reservation for the plane to Teheran was for Friday evening; this meant another day in Rome, which did not disappoint me. Visits to the Piazza del Populo, where the Hotel Rassi used to be, but now there was a business building; to the Forum; to the Colosseum, and the lovely many fountains and then to the Bastienelli Clinic. There I saw the Sister Superior who remembered me and told me that I had just missed Dr. Bastienelli. But she telephoned him and he asked me to come to see him at his home on Via de Vallini. When I went there I was very cordially greeted by the Nestor of Italian surgery, and a great old Roman. He is approaching his 92nd birthday, but is as keen mentally as ever. I said that, the last time I had seen him was in the operating room at the clinic, when he was 85. He said that he had operated until he was 91, 'but my eyes are no longer what they used to be. I now go every day to the clinic to do nothing'. He said that he had been very interested in reading my last paper in the *Annals of Surgery* on the circulation of the living spleen. His American wife had died several years previously so that he was living alone in the museum of a home, with so many beautiful paintings and oriental rugs. There I saw as fine a Samarkand rug as I have ever seen in any museum.

"Rome has not changed at all - the same lovely old pines, the same old Roman wells, the same fountains with their unlimited flow of water, the same great churches and monuments. The traffic in Rome is fantastic. There are few traffic lights, but there are many cross streets, with cars, buses, scooters, and buzzing motor driven bicycles, all going like mad. The scooters and buzzers are the most noisy and hazardous to the pedestrians. Why they do not have more accidents is hard to understand. One has to look four ways on coming to a crossing.

"The people, in general, appear to be prosperous. I saw only two beggars while I was in the city. One of the most frequently seen groups is the very many priests, monks and novitiates in their various kinds of robes. The depreciated lira, like the French franc, is hard to get accustomed to; 2500 lira for a room without a bath, 1800 for a simple meal, 5000 for a suit of clothes.

"November 6th. The stopover in Istanbul was anything but exciting; in a room reserved for transients at two o'clock in the morning. Turkish is a weird language, especially when spelled in the English alphabet, for the Arabic letters have been discarded. The Moslem call to prayer must be a dreadful thing to hear and may be one of the reasons why so few of the modern Turks respond to it.

"We reached Teheran at 10:15, but I saw no one whom I knew at the airport due, I thought, to the misunderstanding about the delay in leaving

Rome. I got through the customs inspection better than I expected. After getting my bags, I asked for a taxi and was led to the worst looking jalopy I had ever seen. The driver seemed to understand my rusty Farsi, or Persian, but he took me through alleys and byways, which made me think that he was giving me the runaround. But he was trying to avoid the closed main highways that had been shut to regular traffic because of the processions that were being held to commemorate the death of the brother of the Shah, who had been killed in a plane accident the day before. This had created a crisis for the Shah, for he has no male heirs and his brother was the Crown Prince, the only other with royal Pehlawi blood.

"My wild Jehu finally deposited me in front of the Bonyadi Iran office where I learned that Mr. Nemazee had left for Paris on the day that I was supposed to arrive in Teheran, when he had planned to meet me before his leaving for Paris. In an hour, Torab Mehra arrived, very distressed that he had not been able to get to the airport to meet me, because of the processions. But he immediately took charge and took me to the travel and visa offices and got me a 'blue card' that is essential for anyone traveling in the country. He had engaged a room at the resort hotel in the suburb Shimron, and drove me there. In the late afternoon he returned and took me to his home where I met his American wife, a former nurse and a Catholic, and their five daughters. Then he and his wife took me to a restaurant where Torab ordered a Persian dinner, Caspian whitefish, shish kababs and a rice pilau, with an Isphahan muskmelon and Turkish coffee for dessert. Back to Shimran, where I got to bed early in preparation for rising at five o'clock to get a 6:30 plane to Isphahan with Torab.

"It had been 58 years since I had been in Iran. I expected and found many changes in the people and buildings, as well as in the traffic in the larger cities, but not so much change in the villages. In them, one sees some advances, such as bicycles, but one sees the same mud houses, primitive methods of agriculture that existed when I was a boy there. But the most remarkable change is in the use of airplanes for traveling between the large cities.

"November 7th. Torab and I took a rather primitive looking plane for Isphahan, but I was reassured when I saw that American pilots flew it. By ten o'clock we reached Isphahan and were driven to the Tourist Hotel, which lived up to its name. But the wonderful sights that we saw that day made up for the deficiencies of the hotel. I had read and heard about the great Maidan, or what is the extensive parade ground, with the palaces and mosques that border the 1,000-4,000 yard quadrangle, as well as of the bazaars that are found near the entrance into the Maidan. But what I saw made the stories about them seem inadequate. On the east and south sides are two of the finest mosques in the world, and on the west side is the palace which Shah Abbas built in the first decade of the 17th century. He also built the two mosques that I mentioned. To the north are the entrances to the bazaars.

"The day I was there they were commemorating the death of the Crown Prince. I heard a loud voice coming from the top of one of the great minarets of the Abbas mosque. Torab said, 'Come up to the front platform of the mosque.' When we got there, I saw a mollah, or priest, sitting before a microphone, chanting a eulogy of the Prince that was transmitted to a loud speaker at the top of the minarets This was another example of the inroads of the West in the East.

"We then went through the bazaars, which seemed endless. As in those in Aleppo and Damascus, the various articles and occupations were shown in different parts of the bazaar - leather goods, dry goods, metal and wood work, carpets, groceries - all had separate areas. The most remarkable spot in the bazaar was a vaulted cavern-like place where two camels were walking in a circle around a platform, pulling two large grindstones that were crushing sesame seeds for the oil contained in them. The camels were blindfolded to prevent their getting dizzy.

"In the afternoon we went to the Armenian suburb of Julfa and saw an unusual Armenian church. In it were astonishing pictures showing the Seven Stations of the Cross. In going there and returning we crossed the famous bridge with its 38 arches, built by the same Shah Abbas. The Isphahanis are much more like the Persians that I used to see in Tabriz.

They wear the same rimless felt hats and wide baggy trousers and cotton woven shoes. Most of the women wear sheet-like coverings, or chuddars, of figured cotton, but no longer wear heavy white veils that covered the heads and faces, as we used to see in Tabriz. There were also the same old smells!

"November 8th. We took another plane for Shiraz the next morning, arriving in Shiraz by mid-morning, where we were met by the professional and nursing staff in a most cordial and genuine welcome. The Hiatts, whom I knew well, drove us to the Saade Hotel, near the Koran entrance to the city. This was an incomparably better hotel than the one in Isphahan, with a fine large garden with a large pool in front of it. After lunch we drove to the hospital where they showed me the different parts; some finished, others not. The third floor was almost finished and is to be used to start the medical and surgical services when the hospital opens on a limited scale.

"During my week's stay I was able to interview every member of the professional and nursing staff which gave me a good idea of how the group felt about the lack of actual caring for patients, and made me realize how important it was to get things started in the hospital, even if it had to be on a very limited scale. This was one of the difficult decisions that I had to make with the members of the staff taking an active part.

"One of the interesting problems of the nursing staff is the indoctrination of the entering class of Moslem girls to our way of thinking of the sick, the care of the male patients, and their dread of having anything to do with the dying or dead patients. They need plenty of training in hygiene and cleanliness. But apparently they are learning fast and are adapting to new ideas."

Footnotes

1. **George A. Brakeley (-)**
   The Treasurer of Princeton University (1941-1952).

2. **Harold Willis Dodds (1889-1980)**
   The 15th president of Princeton University (1933-1957). Dodds led Princeton University through the Great Depression, the Second World War and the post-war period of readjustment.

3. **Charaka Club**
   Founded by Drs. Charles L. Dana, Joseph Colleirs, Fedrick Petterson and Bernard Sachs in 1898, and named after Charaka, a priest and medicine man, to discuss issues surrounding medicine, medical history, literature and even poetry.

4. **Century Club Association**
   Formed in 1847 at a meeting of the Sketch Club, which had been in existence since 1829. One hundred gentlemen engaged or interested in letters and the fine arts had been invited to join in forming the association. Forty-two accepted the invitation and became founders.

5. **Harvey Williams Cushing (1869-1939)**
   A pioneer American neurosurgeon. From 1910 until 1932 he was the Mosley Professor of Surgery and Chairman of the Department at Harvard Medical School, which became the Mecca for neurosurgery. The Cushing's Syndrome and other eponyms carry his name. He was also a medical historian and the biographer of Sir William Osler.

6. **Rudolph Matas (1860-1957)**
   A Professor of Surgery at Tulane University, Louisiana. He was a pioneer in the surgery of the blood vessels, chest and abdomen. His introduction of the suture for the cure of aneurysms won him international fame and caused Sir William Osler to hail him as the "Father of Vascular Surgery" and the "Modern Antyllus". His development of the intravenous drip technique and suction siphonage in abdominal operations brought him honors from colleagues at home and abroad.

7. **Alfred Blalock (1899-1964)**
   The Chairman of Surgery at the Johns Hopkins Hospital (1941-1961). A pioneer cardiovascular surgeon who was the first to operate on coarctation of the aorta.

216

8. **George Whipple (1878-1976)**

A graduate of Johns Hopkins (1905). He is best known for his research in anemia and the physiology and pathology of the liver for which he received the Nobel Prize (1934).

9. **William Mayo (1861-1939)**

A graduate of the University of Michigan School of Medicine (1883). His name is associated with excision of the pylorus; exclusion of the duodenum with posterior gastrojejunostomy; the cure of umbilical hernia; the excision of the rectum with its lymph nodes for cancer. The vein of Mayo is named after him. Along with his brother Charles Mayo (1865-1939), he founded the Mayo Clinic (1915). A prolific surgical aphorist, his aphorisms were collected in: *Aphorisms*. Charles H. Mayo & William. Mayo. Mayo Foundation (1977).

10. **John Finney (1863-1942)**

A graduate of Harvard Medical School (1889). Then appointed by Halsted to the surgical staff of the newly founded Johns Hopkins where he served there until retirement. He is best known for his pyloroplasty (1902). John Finney served as the first president of the American College of Surgeons (1913-1915).

11. **David Cheever (1876-1955)**

One of six generations of Cheevers in direct descent who have graduated from Harvard College. Dr. Cheever graduated from Harvard in 1901 and followed in the footsteps of his distinguished father after whom he was named (the father is best known for his first description of esophagotomy in 1867). The son joined his alma mater in 1913 until he retired as an Emeritus Associate Professor of Surgery in 1939 because of crippling arthritis. He was an active member of the Boston Surgical Society in 1941.

12. **Hindenburg Fire (1937)**

On May of 1937, a German Airship (Zeppelin) "Hindenburg" lifted off the Frankfurt airfield for Lakehurst, NJ on the first of eighteen scheduled visits to North America. Aboard the ship were thirty-six passengers and a crew of sixty-one. Just before landing the airship burst into massive flames at an altitude of 200 feet. Out of the 97 on board, 48 died in the accident.

Chapter Twenty-one

Epilogue

1962 - 1963

September 21, 1962. After almost three years I am resuming this rather casual story of my doings. After living at the Nasman Club for six months, I moved to a one floor apartment on Stanworth Lane, a block east of the apartment where mum and I spent our last days together. The family to whom I had rented the apartment, furnished, left it in inexcusably bad condition, even breaking some of the Venetian glass that we had tried to use only on special occasions. How different from the way mum always left a house or apartment spotless when we moved out!

My one floor apartment had been repainted and was spotless. The problem was what to put in and what to leave out, for room was limited to a living room, very small kitchen, bathroom and two bedrooms, one of which I used as a study. So a good share of the furniture and the books that we had in the two-room apartment had to go into storage. It took ten days to set the place in order, and gave occupation during a hot August.

Much of the last two years have been spent in writing. First the monograph; *The Role of the Nestorians and the Moslems in the History of Medicine*. I had a sense of obligation to the American Societies of Oriental Research to write this and have it published. But it has not much selling value, except to those interested in the history of medicine. I took it to two large publishing houses without success, but it is now in the hands of the Bollingel foundation, interested in the Near and Middle East. I have some assurance that they will accept it [1].

A year ago I got interested in writing *The Story of Wound Healing and Wound Repair*, a subject that I was engaged in during my active years in surgery and one that I had studied in reading the history of medicine. After finishing this work, I sent it to the Thomas Publishers and was surprised to have it accepted immediately. They hope to have it published by Christmas [2].

The third book, which I have recently finished, on *The Evolution of Surgery in the United States* was also sent to the Thomas people. I informed them that I was writing it and, to my great surprise, they accepted it sight unseen, and sent me a contract to be signed which I did before they could change their mind. I had been asked to give a lecture on that subject at the Albany Medical College in November. In preparing this lecture I found so much more of interest than I could include in a hour lecture that I decided to write a book on the subject [3].

It is not well known that surgery in our country, beginning with the advent of the colonists, had to be done largely by untrained people, for very few doctors, if any, came over with the Virginians and the Pilgrims. Much of the care of the sick for the first century of the colonies was done by the administrators and the clergymen. But as the towns and cities developed, the surgeons settled in the urban areas and the young men wanting to study medicine and surgery, studied as apprentices for one to three years before starting to practice. Later some of the well-to-do young men went to London or Edinburgh to study, and a few of them, after training in the British medical centers, returned and started medical schools in this country. The first was in Philadelphia, the second in Columbia College in New York, the third was at Harvard in Boston, and the fourth in Dartmouth College in Hanover, New Hampshire.

Some of the well-trained surgeons settled not only in the cities of the eastern seaboard, but went to the outlying settlements in what later became Kentucky and Ohio. There they did some very remarkable surgery, with little help, no anesthesia, on kitchen tables in primitive huts. Ephraim McDowell did the first abdominal operation, in 1809, on a woman with a very large ovarian cyst. She had to ride three days on horseback to get from her home to McDowell's surgery some 60 miles away. This operation was successful and the woman lived another thirty years. I must stop, or I will be copying the book!

In February of last year, Bumps came to Princeton and has been living in the apartment with me, spending much of his time in writing. His first book was called *Three Traitors* and had to do with Benedict Arnold, Aaron Burr and Wilkinson, the latter less well known, but the worst of the three. This book had to do with the period before, during, and after the Revolution. It seemed to me to be a good piece of writing. He had the advantage of using the Firestone Library here in the university. The book is in the hands of an agent, and he hopes it will be published soon [4]. Meanwhile he is writing a book on the experiences he and others in his squadron on the Essex had in the Pacific during World War II. Some of these experiences were very amusing, others tragic, both well told.

In May of 1962 I went to Washington to attend the meeting of the American Surgical Association. While there I had two attacks of cardiac, or heart pain. It made me realize that I should return to Princeton without delay. When I reached home, I found that my friend and physician, DeWitt Smith, was recovering from an operation at the Neurological Institute in New York, so I went to his associate. He took an electrocardiogram and, after examining it, told me that he knew I would want to go to the Presbyterian Hospital in New York. He called an ambulance and said I should go to the Harkness immediately. He also called my friend, Howard Bruenn [5], the cardiologist at the Presbyterian. So, without delay, I was taken to the Harkness and spent the next six weeks there in a good room; four weeks in bed and two weeks with increased walking. Every other day I had electrocardiograms and blood coagulation tests, and was given as thorough a work-up as could be done anywhere. Certainly the doctors and nurses could not have been kinder or more solicitous. The last two weeks, after the "no visitors" sign was removed, I was able to see so many of my old friends in and out of the hospital.

The night before I was to leave the hospital, I was allowed to attend a dinner at the Union Club for the seven surgeons who had retired, during the previous fifteen months; four of them were my first residents. This certainly dated me. But it was a delightful informal party, with no set speeches and a circulating lot of some 150 diners. Wilder Penfield was there from Montreal. He had recently returned from a neurological consultation on one of the top communists in China, very much as he had done for one of the leading astrophysicists in Moscow the year before.

My physicians have given me a small bottle of nitroglycerine tablets to take if I have any recurrence of cardiac pain, but I have not had to use them, though I carry them in my pocket at all times. It has been a talisman. But I know that I am living on borrowed time, and am ready to go whenever the time comes. Life has been so interesting, with so many precious memories and good friends. I have had more than my share of good health, and this is one of the things I am most grateful for.

Footnotes

1. Published in one edition in 1967. Princeton University Press, Princeton, New Jersey.

2. Published in one edition in 1963. Charles C. Thomas, Springfield, IL.

3. Published in one edition in 1963. Charles C. Thomas, Springfield, IL.

4. Not clear if it was ever published.

5. **Howard Bruenn (1905-1995)**
    A Columbia College graduate who later became a physician and cardiologist to President Franklin D. Roosevelt during the President's last year of life.